THE COMPLETE GUIDE TO

NATURAL VITAMINS

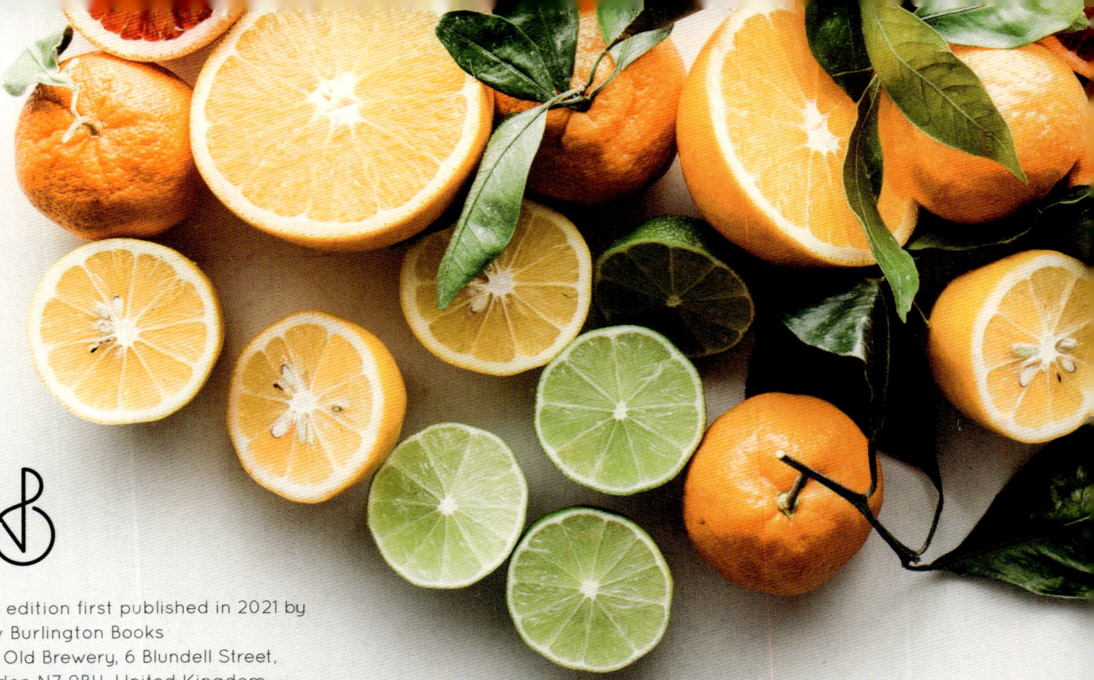

This edition first published in 2021 by
New Burlington Books
The Old Brewery, 6 Blundell Street,
London N7 9BH, United Kingdom

ISBN 978-0-85762-991-3

Conceived, designed, and produced by The Bright Press, an imprint of
The Quarto Group
The Old Brewery, 6 Blundell Street, London N7 9BH, United Kingdom
T (0) 20 7700 6700
www.QuartoKnows.com

Publisher: James Evans
Editorial Director: Isheeta Mustafi
Managing Editor: Jacqui Sayers
Project Editor: Anna Southgate
Art Director: James Lawrence
Designer: Studio Noel
Picture Research: Studio Noel
Reviewed by Katie Chapman, MS, RD
Editorial Assistant: Chloë Porter

Cover images from Shutterstock: Front: Flaffy; Back left: Katrinshine; back center: MasterQ; back right: Pinkyone

Manufactured in China

10 9 8 7 6 5 4 3 2 1

While every care has been taken in presenting this material, the information is not intended to replace professional nutritional advice; it should not be used as a guide for self-treatment or self-diagnosis. Neither the author nor the publisher may be held responsible for any type of damage or harm caused by the use or misuse of information in this book and any person with a condition requiring medical attention should consult a qualified medical practitioner or therapist.

THE COMPLETE GUIDE TO NATURAL VITAMINS FROM FOOD AND SUPPLEMENTS

Lizzie Streit, MS, RDN, LD

[CONTENTS]

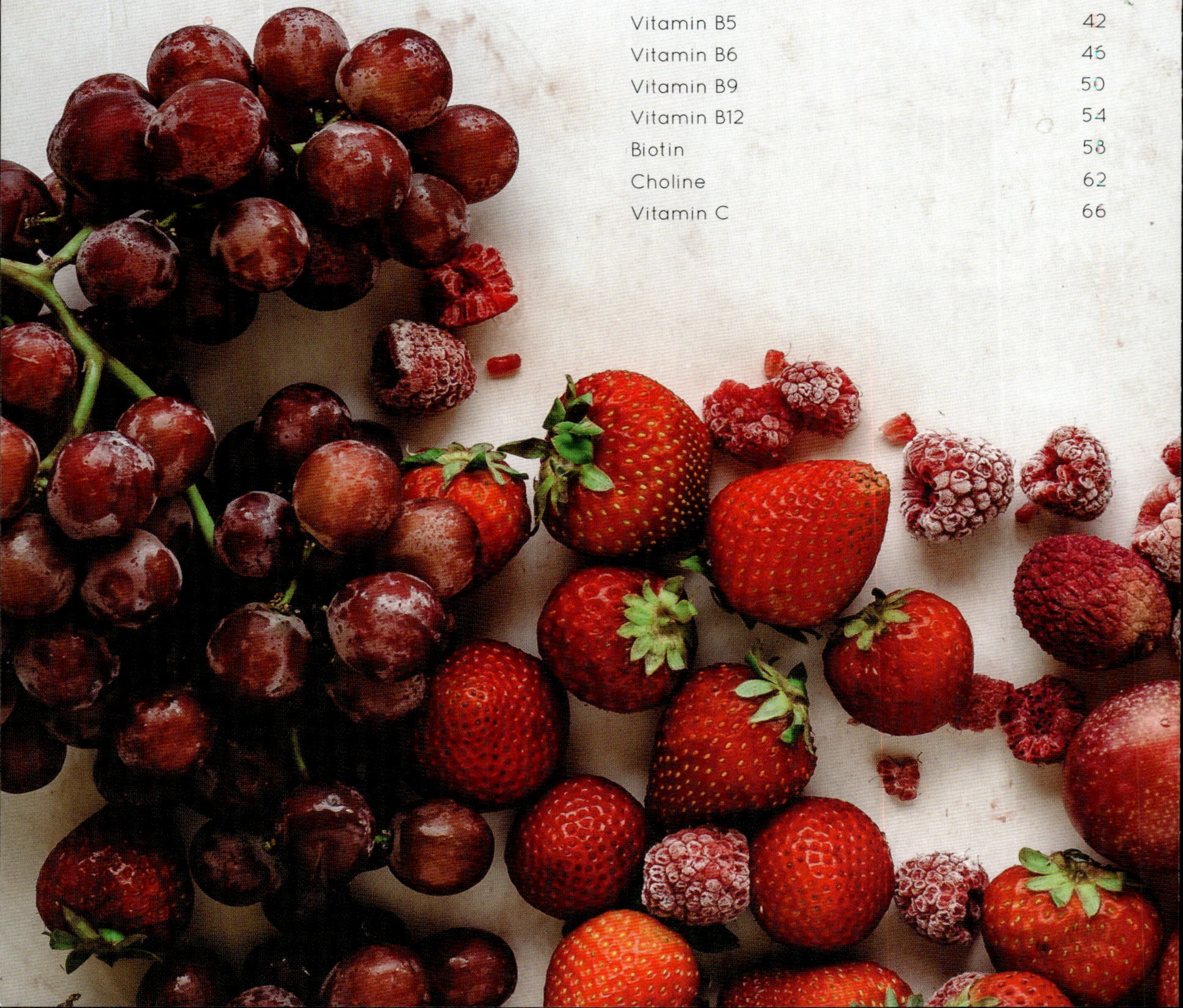

PART TWO:

MINERALS 70

PART THREE:

VITAMINS, MINERALS, AND YOU 132

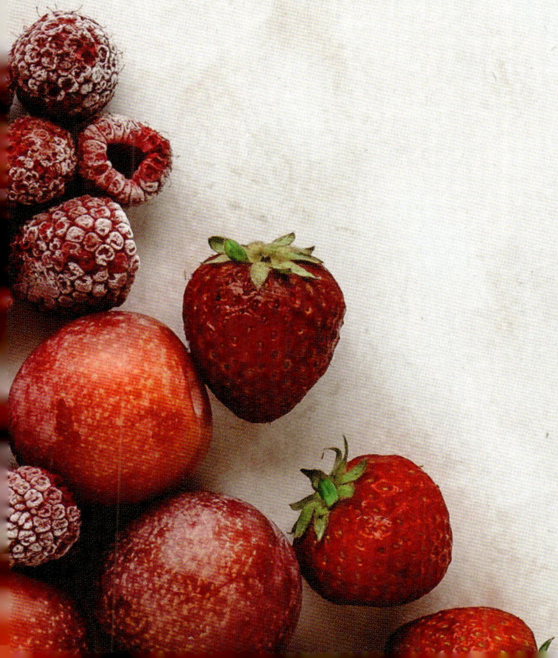

[INTRODUCTION]

Welcome to your complete guide to vitamins and minerals! Perhaps you picked up this book to gain a better understanding of what these nutrients do in the body and how you can get enough of them. Maybe you follow a special diet and want to prevent deficiencies, or you want to know if, when, and how you should take supplements. No matter your reason for reading this book, you'll learn everything you need to know about the fundamentals of vitamins and minerals on the following pages.

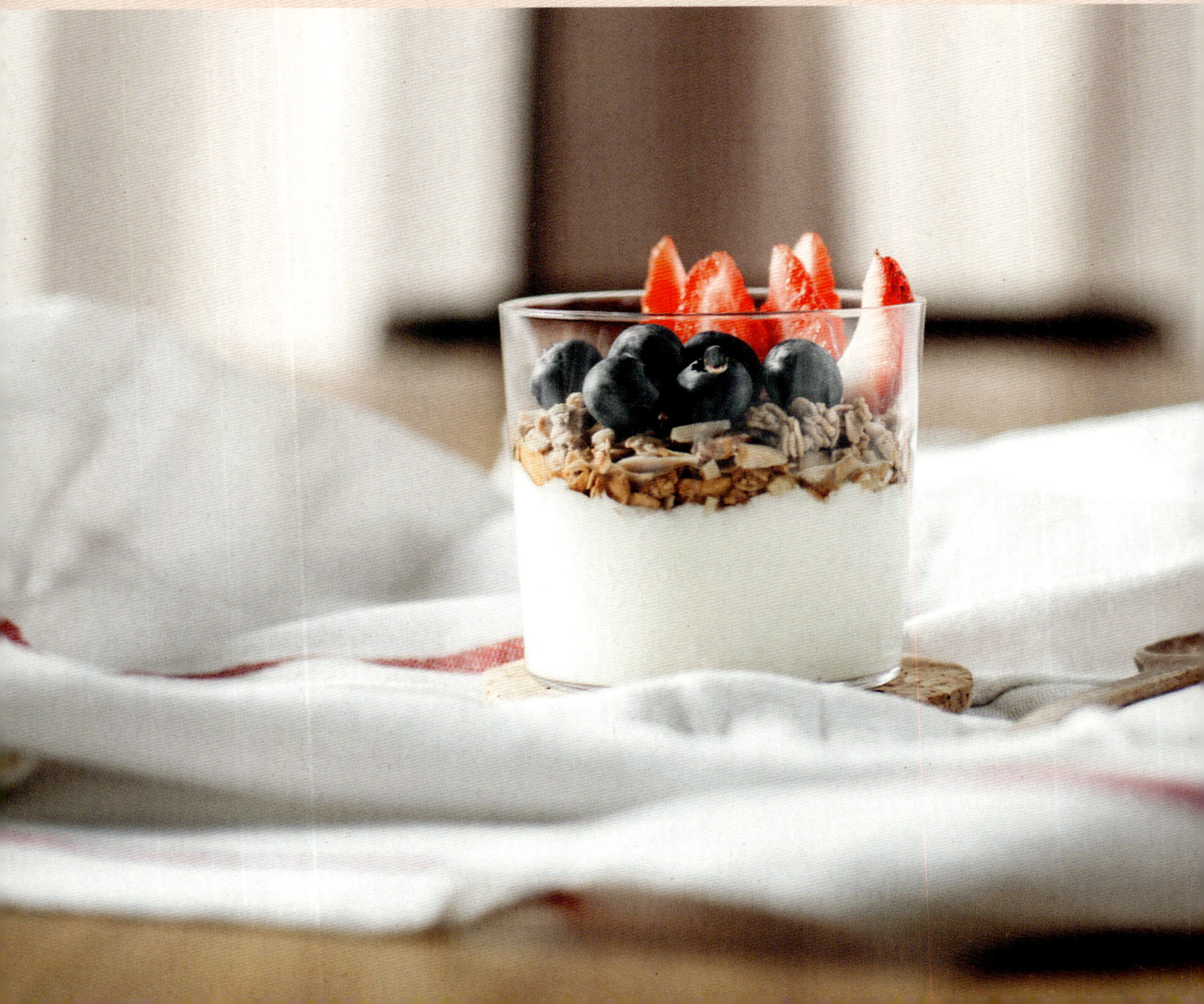

UNDERSTANDING VITAMINS AND MINERALS

Vitamins and minerals are micronutrients. They're needed in fairly small amounts but are vital for human health and have very important functions in the body. This book covers the essential vitamins and minerals—that is, the ones that the body can't make itself or doesn't produce in adequate amounts. While it is "essential" to get these 30 nutrients from dietary sources, it should also be noted that getting too much of any one of them may do more harm than good. In addition to providing information about the main functions, food sources, and signs of deficiency for each nutrient, this guide includes points of interest about toxicity and the safety of taking vitamin and mineral supplements.

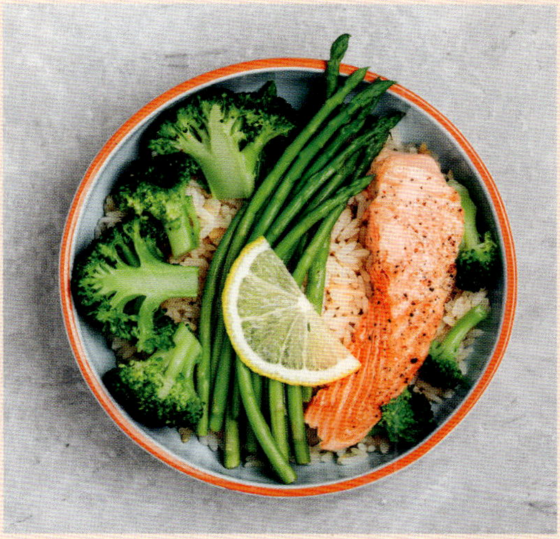

Salmon is one of very few dietary sources of vitamin D; broccoli and asparagus contain folate (vitamin B9).

Vitamins are organic compounds, meaning they contain carbon and can be broken down or changed by heat, light, or air. Thus, cooking and storage techniques can decrease the vitamin content of foods. The two main groups of vitamins are fat-soluble, which include vitamins A, D, E, and K, and water-soluble, made up of the eight B vitamins, the compound choline, and vitamin C. Water-soluble vitamins can dissolve in water, are readily absorbed, and tend to be easily eliminated through urine when you consume too much of them. Fat-soluble vitamins, on the other hand, do not dissolve in water and can be stored in fat tissues. Some fat-soluble vitamins may therefore accumulate in toxic amounts in the body when consumed in excess, usually as a result of over-supplementation and not from dietary intake.

Minerals are inorganic compounds that cannot be changed by heat, light, or air. Plant foods, fish, and other animals absorb minerals from soil and/or water. Since heat does not break down minerals in food, cooking will not affect them in the same away as it impacts vitamin content. However, some minerals can still be lost from food via juices that leak out during cooking. The minerals are divided into two groups: major and trace, which are needed in relatively larger and smaller amounts, respectively. The major minerals include calcium, chloride, magnesium, phosphorus, potassium, sodium, and sulfur. Chromium, copper, fluoride, iodine, iron, manganese, molybdenum, selenium, and zinc are the trace minerals.

Plain yogurt is one of the top calcium-rich foods.

REQUIREMENTS AND GUIDELINES

The Dietary Reference Intakes (DRIs), or the reference values used for recommended nutrient intakes, are included for each vitamin and mineral. The Food and Nutrition Board at the Institute of Medicine for the National Academies establishes these reference values for healthy people. You will see the following DRIs throughout this book:

- **Recommended Dietary Allowance (RDA):** The RDA refers to the average level of nutrient intake per day that's sufficient to meet the needs of up to 98% of healthy individuals.
- **Adequate Intake (AI):** The AI, or the level of nutrient intake that's assumed to be sufficient for nutritional adequacy, is established when there's not enough evidence to recommend an RDA.
- **Tolerable Upper Intake Level (UL):** The UL indicates the maximum daily intake of a nutrient that is unlikely to cause adverse health effects. Not every nutrient has an established UL.

The established reference values vary by age and gender. Men and women often require different amounts of nutrients from one another, as do pregnant and lactating women. The values for some nutrients may also change for older adults. If there are no variations in nutrient needs across age groups, the values are listed for men and women, which refers to adults who are 19 years of age and older.

It's important to keep in mind that these values refer to the nutrient needs of an average healthy person. As you will learn in this book, certain medical conditions, phases of the life cycle, and special diets may impact nutrient needs. While the values are a good starting point for assessing nutritional intake, they may not be the most accurate benchmark for some individuals. If you have concerns about your vitamin and mineral requirements or intake, consult with a physician and registered dietitian.

UNDER 18s

Values for children are not included in this book. Generally, infants and children need smaller amounts of nutrients compared to adults. To learn about the needs of individuals under 18 years of age, you should refer to the National Institutes of Health (NIH) consumer fact sheets for each vitamin and mineral.

MAKING THE RIGHT FOOD CHOICES DURING PREGNANCY AND LACTATION

Each vitamin and mineral includes suggested nutrient intakes for pregnant and lactating women. However, not all of the foods listed in the "Common Food Sources" are recommended during pregnancy. Pregnant and lactating women should follow the advice of their health care providers before including any of the recommended foods.

Throughout this book, you'll find beautiful, inspiring food images to help you find ways to include a good variety of nutrients in your diet every day.

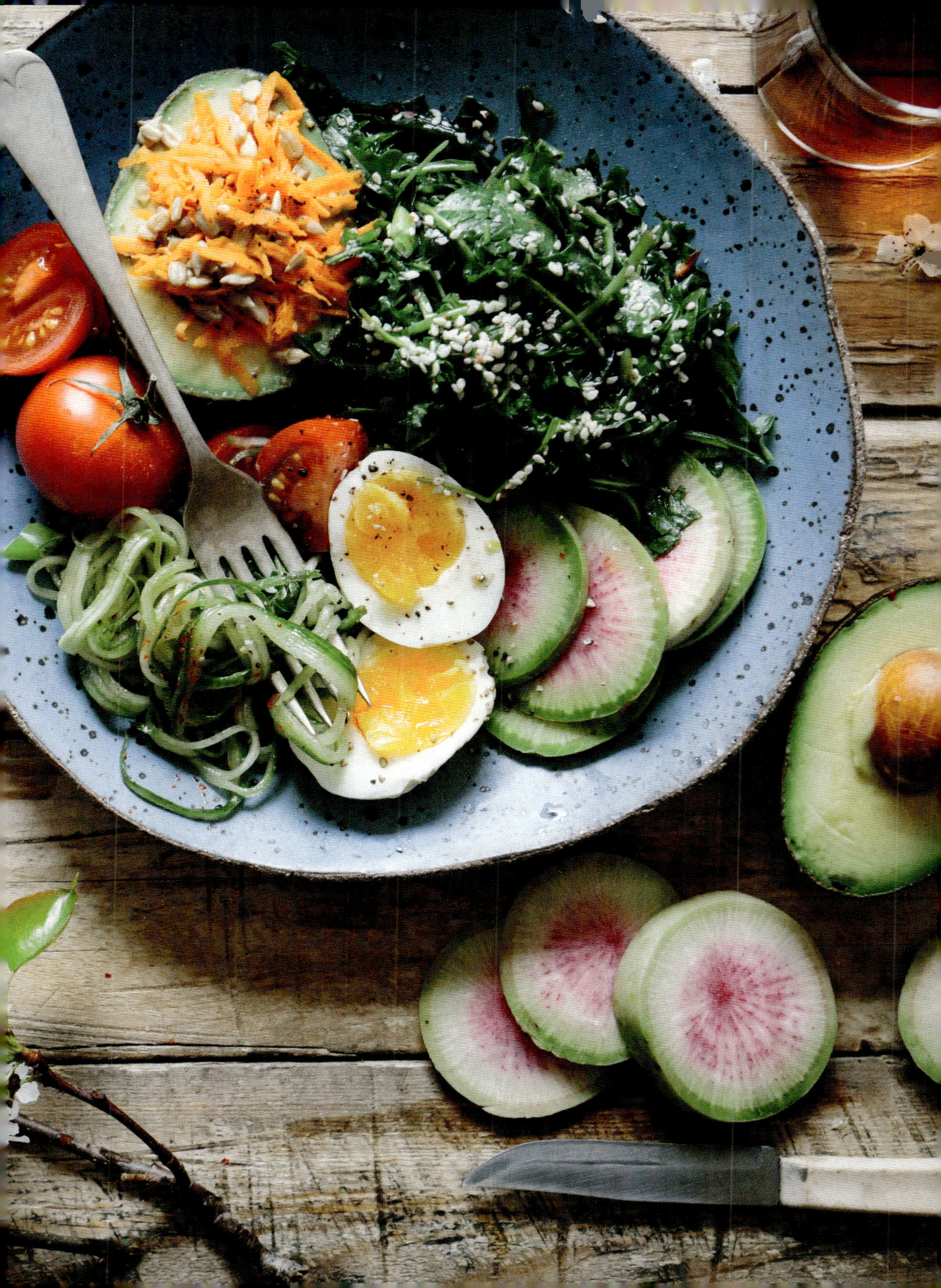

[HOW TO USE THIS BOOK]

Part One of this book covers the essential vitamins, starting with the fat-soluble vitamins and continuing with the water-soluble vitamins and choline (a vitamin-like compound). Part Two looks at the major minerals before introducing the trace minerals. The last section of the book, Part Three, includes a selection of feature spreads about applying your knowledge of vitamins and minerals to your everyday diet.

Each vitamin or mineral section includes the following topics:

RDAs/AIs: These are listed at the start of each entry.

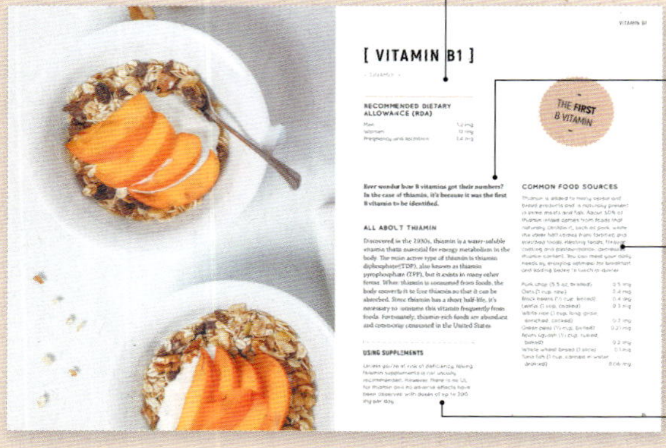

Introduction: Explores the history of each nutrient and the main points of interest about functions, food sources, and deficiency.

Food Sources: Includes some of the best food sources for the nutrient, as well as options for lesser-known ones.

Using Supplements: Considers if and when supplements may be useful or necessary. If there is an established UL for a nutrient or concerns about toxicity, it's discussed here.

Role in the Body: Examines the main functions of each vitamin and mineral in the body and their roles in disease prevention or management.

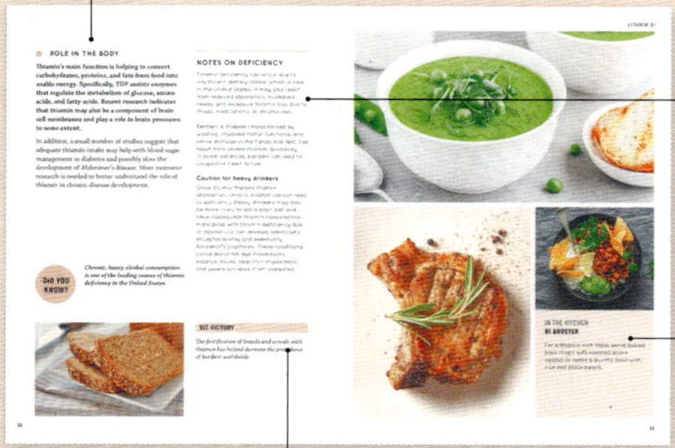

Notes on Deficiency: Looks at the prevalence of deficiency, signs and symptoms, and at-risk groups.

In the Kitchen: Recipe ideas help you get enough nutrients in delicious and easy ways.

Vit/Mineral Tips: Offer factors that impact nutrient absorption and how to boost intake via the kitchen.

The final pages of the book are devoted to common questions and interests when it comes to vitamins and minerals. Topics include how nutrients work together in the body, antioxidants, nutrition through the life cycle, and common supplements, among others. The book ends with a sample weekly meal plan to help you plan balanced, nutrient-dense meals.

ENRICHED AND FORTIFIED FOODS

Some of the foods listed in the "Common Food Sources" may be identified as enriched or fortified. Fortification refers to the process of adding nutrients to a food that it does not naturally contain, such as vitamin D in milk. Enrichment is the term for replacing nutrients that were lost during food processing—the B vitamins in enriched breads and pastas, for example. A version of a food that's not fortified or enriched may no longer be a good source of a certain nutrient. For example, calcium-fortified orange juice is a good source of calcium, but orange juice that's not fortified is not as high in calcium. Generally, fortified and enriched foods are better sources of nutrients than supplements.

APPLYING REFERENCE VALUES TO YOUR DIET

The RDA or AI for a certain nutrient refers to the suggested average daily intake. However, you don't have to exactly meet these recommendations every day. Instead, focus on your weekly intake of each nutrient, and aim to eat the required amount as part of a more varied diet. First, calculate the weekly intake needed for a nutrient—vitamin A, for example—by multiplying the RDA by seven (for the days of the week):

- 700 mcg (the RDA) x 7 = 4,900 mcg of vitamin A needed per week

Then you can asses how much a food source, such as one sweet potato, contributes to your weekly requirement of that nutrient. You can then work out how much more of the food source you need to eat in order to make up the full requirement:

- 4,900 mcg – 1403 mcg (1 sweet potato) = 3497 mcg of vitamin A left to meet
- 3497 mcg ÷ 1403 mcg = 2.5 sweet potatoes left to eat

Sweet potatoes are included here for the sake of the example but, of course, it's best to eat a variety of foods to meet your nutrient needs. You can perform these same calculations with other foods listed under vitamin A, and keep in mind that there are many foods that are good sources of a nutrient that are not listed. Browse MedicalNewsToday.com, Healthline.com, Hsph.Harvard.edu, or WedMD.com for other food sources. Once you have identified some, use Pinterest or Google to search for recipes.

When using the food lists, think of the foods and their nutrient contents as a guide instead of definitive amounts. The amount of a vitamin or mineral that a food contains may differ based on growing conditions, food processing, and preparation techniques.

PART ONE:
VITAMINS

This section provides an overview of the 13 essential vitamins and the vitamin-like nutrient choline. You'll learn how each vitamin acts in the body and what happens during deficiency.

The information here will help you start to assess your vitamin intake and status. You'll also find tips for putting the info to use in the kitchen, bringing you one step closer to a more balanced, nutritionally complete diet. Simply bookmark your favorite pages to return to when you need a refresher.

Getting vitamins through your diet is best, since taking too many supplements can be dangerous in some cases. Be sure to discuss any concerns about micronutrients with your health care provider.

DID YOU KNOW?

Meeting vitamin needs from foods, but not supplements, has been linked to longevity. Studies show that taking vitamins in pill form does not have the same beneficial effects as eating a wide variety of healthful, vitamin-rich foods.

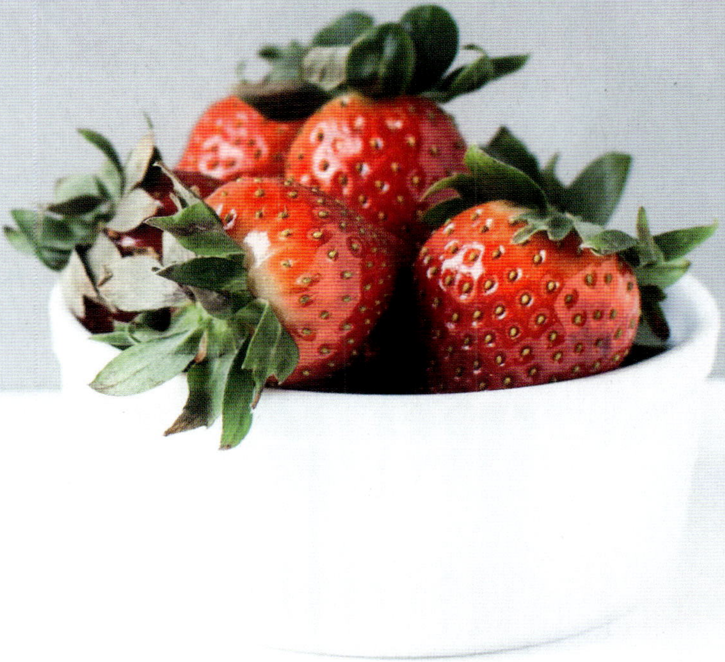

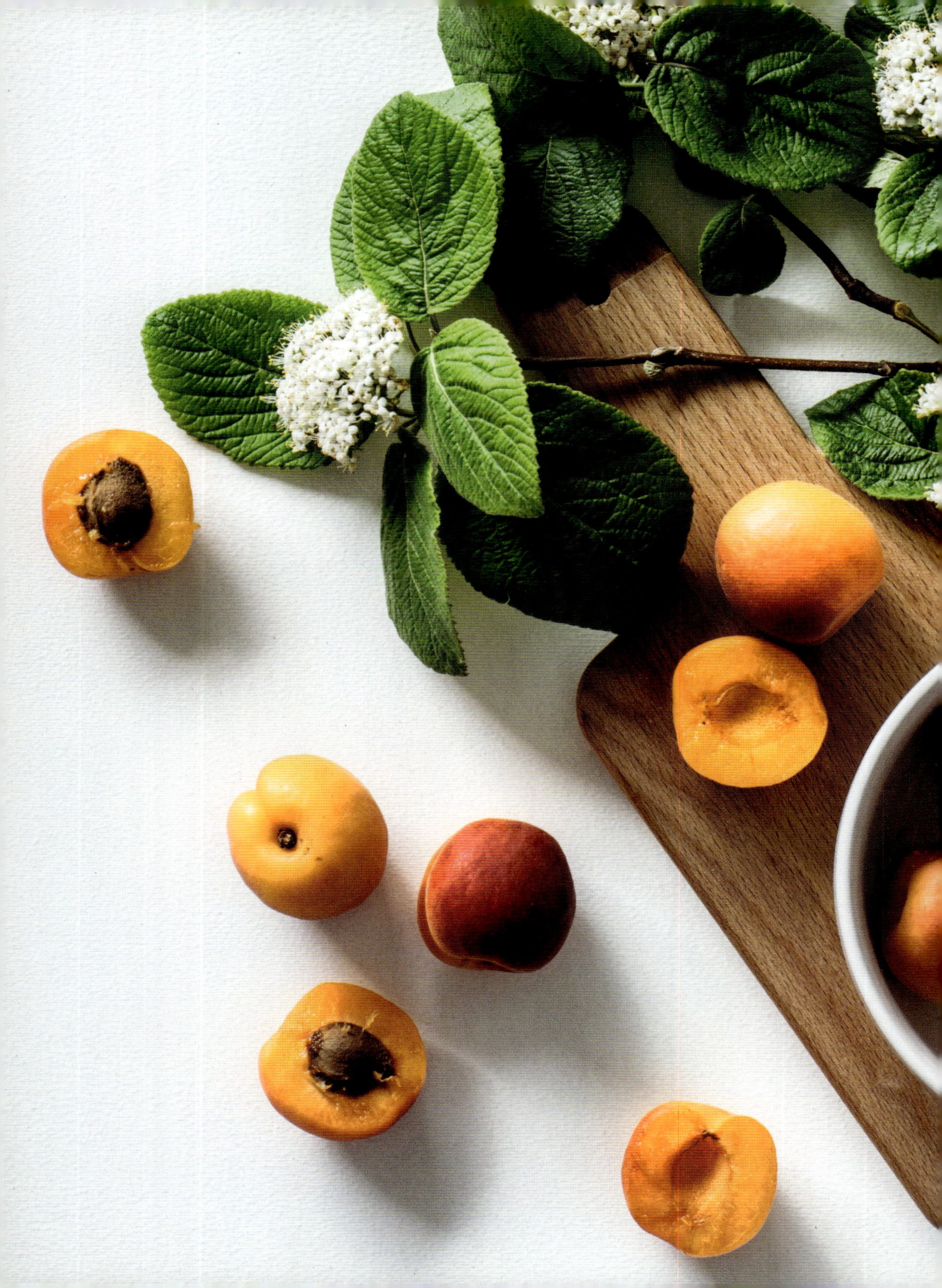

[VITAMIN A]

- RETINOL -

THE **VISION** AID

RECOMMENDED DIETARY ALLOWANCE (RDA)

Men	900 mcg RAE
Women	700 mcg RAE
Pregnancy (up to 18 years)	750 mcg RAE
Pregnancy (19+ years)	770 mcg RAE
Lactation (up to 18 years)	1,200 mcg RAE
Lactation (19+ years)	1,300 mcg RAE

RAE: retinol activity equivalents

If you've been told to eat more carrots for good eyesight, then you know that vitamin A plays a vital role in eye health, among other functions.

ALL ABOUT RETINOL

This vitamin includes two groups of fat-soluble compounds: preformed vitamin A (retinol and retinyl esters) and provitamin A carotenoids. Preformed vitamin A is found in animal products, while carotenoids mostly come from plant foods. The best-known provitamin A carotenoid, beta-carotene, is responsible for the orange color of carrots and sweet potatoes.

Provitamin A carotenoids must be converted to retinol, an active form of vitamin A, in the body. The RDA for vitamin A is therefore given in retinol activity equivalents (RAE), which accounts for the different activities of retinol and provitamin A carotenoids. The good news is, since carotenoids are converted to retinol, anyone following a vegan or vegetarian diet can meet their needs from plants.

COMMON FOOD SOURCES

Sources of preformed vitamin A in the diet include liver, fish and fish oils, and milk. Provitamin carotenoids are found in a variety of fruits and vegetables, including carrots, apricots, spinach, pumpkin, and broccoli. Just one baked sweet potato with skin will give you enough vitamin A for two days.

Beef liver (1 oz, braised)	2,650 mcg
Sweet potato (1 medium, baked, with skin)	1,403 mcg
Carrots (½ cup, raw)	459 mcg
Spinach (2 cups, raw)	282 mcg
Whole milk (1 cup)	112 mcg
Salmon (1 medium fillet, steamed/poached)	79 mcg
Papaya (1 cup)	78 mcg
Apricots (10 halves, dried)	63 mcg

USING SUPPLEMENTS

High doses of preformed vitamin A from supplements can be toxic and are rarely recommended. Always check with your health care provider before trying one. (See also, Vitamin A Toxicity, page 16.)

ROLE IN THE BODY

A necessary nutrient for good eyesight and immune health, vitamin A has many important roles in the body. The retina, as it is aptly named, requires vitamin A to function normally. Not getting enough vitamin A can lead to poor night vision and the formation of small spots in the white part of the eyes, known as Bitot's spots.

Even before birth, vitamin A is vital for the development of the eyes, heart, lungs, and other important organs. Vitamin A also regulates immune cells, helping the body resist infection and disease, and works as an antioxidant to fight cell damage.

NOTES ON DEFICIENCY

Vitamin A deficiency is rare in the United States, but can be common in developing countries where communities have limited access to food sources of this nutrient. Children and pregnant women are especially at risk in these areas.

Symptoms of vitamin A deficiency include night blindness and weakened resistance to infection. Since deficiency is highly unlikely if you live in the United States, taking vitamin A supplements is not usually recommended.

VITAMIN A TOXICITY

The body regulates the conversion of provitamin A, so toxicity is unlikely to develop from provitamin A carotenoids. Nevertheless, as a fat-soluble compound, extra vitamin A can accumulate in the liver. Unless you eat copious amounts of animal liver, it's most common to develop vitamin A toxicity from supplements rather than food. In high doses, preformed vitamin A supplements can cause potentially harmful side effects and even lead to death in rare cases.

Pregnant women should be careful with vitamin A supplements, as excess preformed vitamin A has been linked to birth defects. If your prenatal vitamin contains vitamin A, make sure it's from provitamin A carotenoids. Some prenatal vitamins may have a mixture of provitamin A carotenoids and retinyl esters. Be sure to check the label and discuss supplements with your physician before taking them.

The toxic upper limit (UL) for preformed vitamin A is 3,000 mcg for men and women over 18 years of age. If you are curious how much preformed vitamin A versus provitamin A carotenoids a supplement contains, check the label to see the breakdown.

DID YOU KNOW?

Because of its role in immunity, vitamin A was called "the anti-infective vitamin" during research studies in the 1920s.

VIT TIPS

Eating foods that contain vitamin A with a source of fat helps with absorption. Try drizzling cooked spinach with olive oil or add avocado to a baked sweet potato.

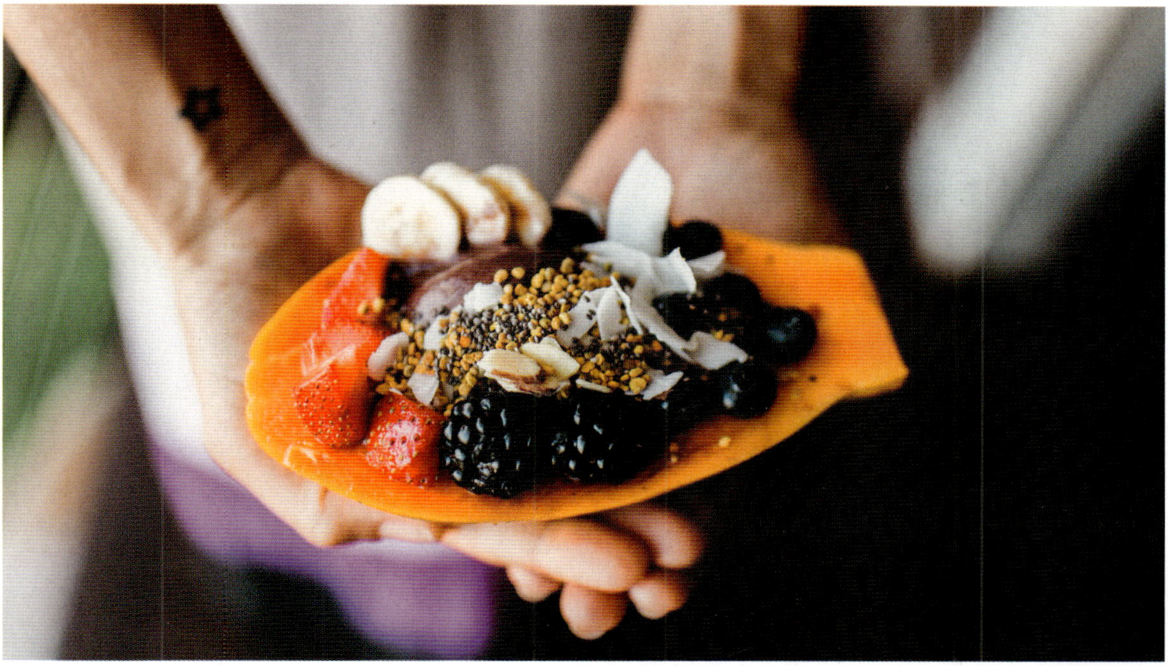

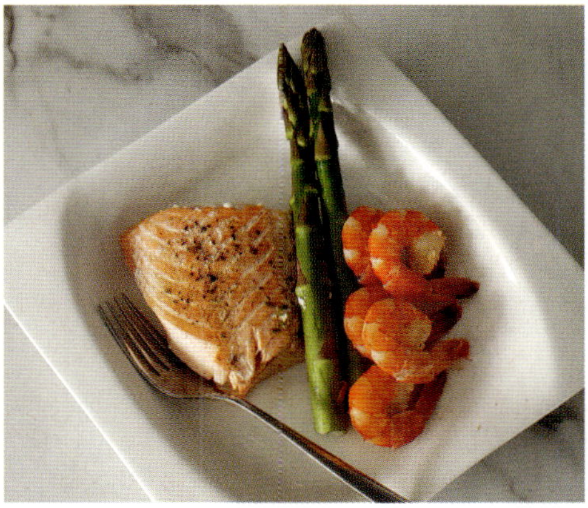

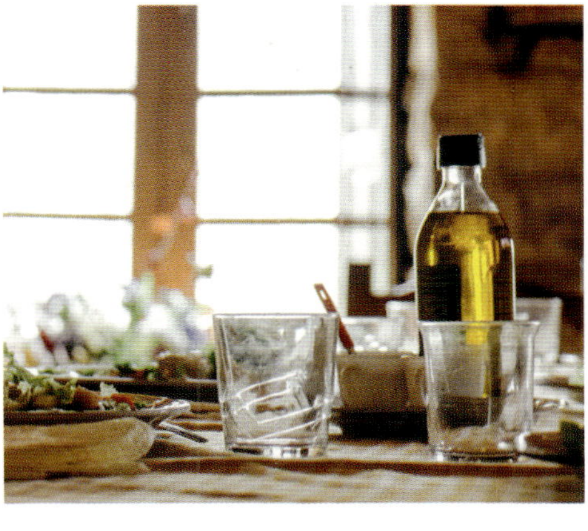

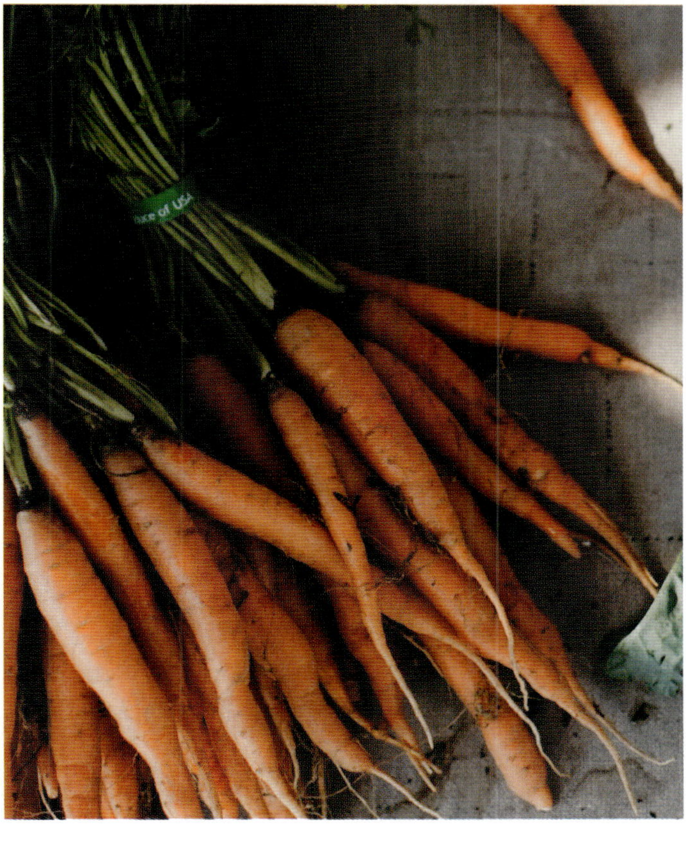

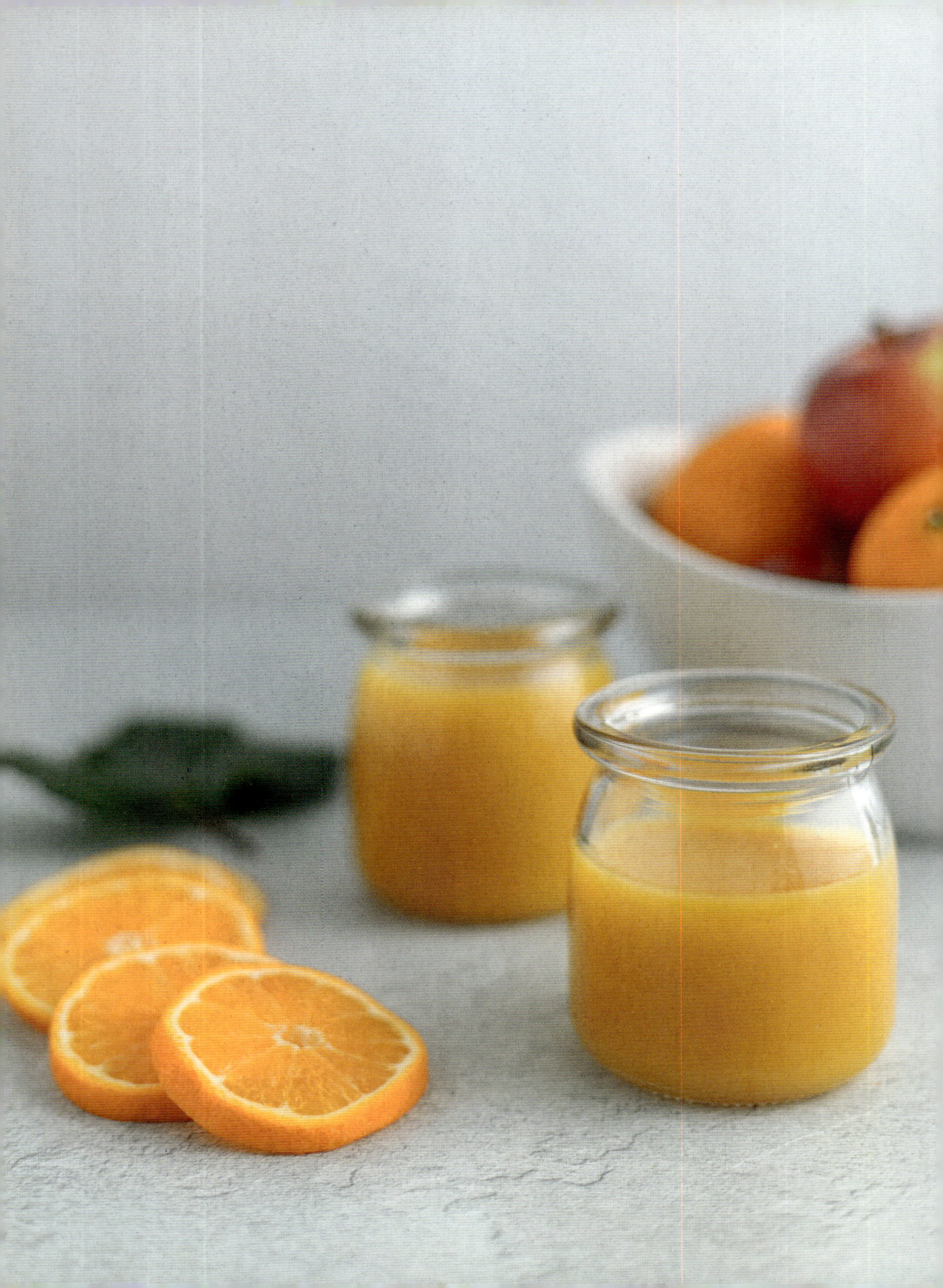

[VITAMIN D]

- CALCIFEROL -

THE **SUNSHINE** VITAMIN

RECOMMENDED DIETARY ALLOWANCE (RDA)

Men and women:	
(18–70 years)	15 mcg (600 IU)
(70+ years)	20 mcg (800 IU)
Pregnancy and lactation	15 mcg (600 IU)

Soaking up the sun isn't just good for the soul. It's also necessary for the synthesis of vitamin D in the body. When sunlight hits the skin, it triggers the production of vitamin D and the metabolism of this nutrient into its active form by the liver and kidneys.

ALL ABOUT CALCIFEROL

Vitamin D, also known as calciferol, is a fat-soluble vitamin that acts similarly to a hormone. It signals important processes in the body, including the regulation of blood calcium and phosphorus levels and bone mineralization.

The best way to meet the RDA for vitamin D is to get 10 to 30 minutes of sun on bare skin, preferably around midday, several days a week. Individuals with darker skin may need longer exposure, while those who have fair skin or a higher risk of skin cancer should be more cautious. In these instances, it's important to meet recommended vitamin D intakes from food or supplement sources in addition to, or instead of, the sun. The current RDAs for this nutrient assume limited sun exposure. Amounts of vitamin D in foods or supplements are either listed as micrograms (mcg) or international units (IU), with one IU equaling 0.025 mcg.

COMMON FOOD SOURCES

Vitamin D exists in two forms in food and supplements: vitamin D2, found in mushrooms exposed to UV light and some fortified foods, and vitamin D3, which exists in fish and egg yolks. However, few foods are natural sources. Consuming a tablespoon of cod liver oil a few times a week will meet the RDA.

Cod liver oil (1 tbsp)	34 mcg
Sockeye salmon (3 oz, cooked)	12 mcg
Mushrooms (½ cup, raw, exposed to UV light)	9 mcg
2% milk (1 cup, fortified)	3 mcg
Orange juice (½ cup, fortified)	1.25 mcg
Tuna fish (3 oz, canned in water, drained)	1 mcg
Egg yolk (1 large)	0.9 mcg

USING SUPPLEMENTS

The use of vitamin D supplements is common. Most contain vitamin D3, in doses ranging from 400 to 2,000 IU. The upper limit (UL) is 100 mcg (4,000 IU) per day for adults. (See also, Notes on Deficiency, page 20, and page 151.)

ROLE IN THE BODY

Vitamin D is essential for promoting optimal bone health by regulating the blood levels of calcium and phosphorus. The active form of vitamin D increases intestinal absorption and maintains adequate levels of these two nutrients, which is necessary for bone growth and remodeling.

Many cells also have vitamin D receptors (VDR) that bind to vitamin D. As a result, vitamin D plays a role in regulating immune system cells as well as the cells that release insulin in the pancreas. Finally, vitamin D may decrease the synthesis of renin, a protein that's involved in increasing blood pressure. The potential roles of vitamin D in boosting immunity, regulating blood sugar, and maintaining healthy blood pressure continue to be the focus of a growing body of scientific studies.

VIT TIPS

Did you know, if you get a lot of sun exposure in the summer, your body can store vitamin D for the winter months? Given that most people work indoors, however, and since excess sun exposure is linked to skin cancer, it's difficult for the average person to benefit from this.

DID YOU KNOW?

At latitudes above 37°N (north of Indianapolis and Denver, for example), there is not enough sunlight from November through March to produce sufficient vitamin D in the skin.

NOTES ON DEFICIENCY

Having deficient or insufficient blood levels of vitamin D is thought to be common, with some research estimating that more than 40% of US adults are deficient. Still, the best ways to evaluate vitamin D status and the prevalence of deficiency remain up for debate.

Other studies suggest that 18% of people over one year of age in the United States are at risk of vitamin D insufficiency. Experts generally consider blood levels below 30 nmol/L as deficient and between 30 to 49 nmol/L as insufficient. If you are deficient in vitamin D, taking supplements is the best way to boost blood levels. However, you should discuss your options with your health care provider and have your blood vitamin D levels monitored, as it is possible to develop vitamin D toxicity from supplements but not from sun exposure. See Spotlight on Vitamin D, page 151.

Who's at risk?

Groups at risk of vitamin D deficiency include exclusively breastfed infants, since human milk does not provide enough of this nutrient, and older adults, as the skin loses its ability to synthesize vitamin D over time. People with limited sun exposure, dark skin, and fat malabsorption issues may also be at risk.

What are the symptoms?

Vitamin D deficiency often manifests as bone issues and diseases. Children who are deficient in vitamin D may develop rickets, marked by soft bones and bowed arms and legs. While rickets is rare in the United States, thanks to the fortification of milk in the 1930s, it has been reported in African, Middle Eastern, and Asian countries. Adults with severe vitamin D deficiency may develop weak, soft bones and a condition known as osteomalacia.

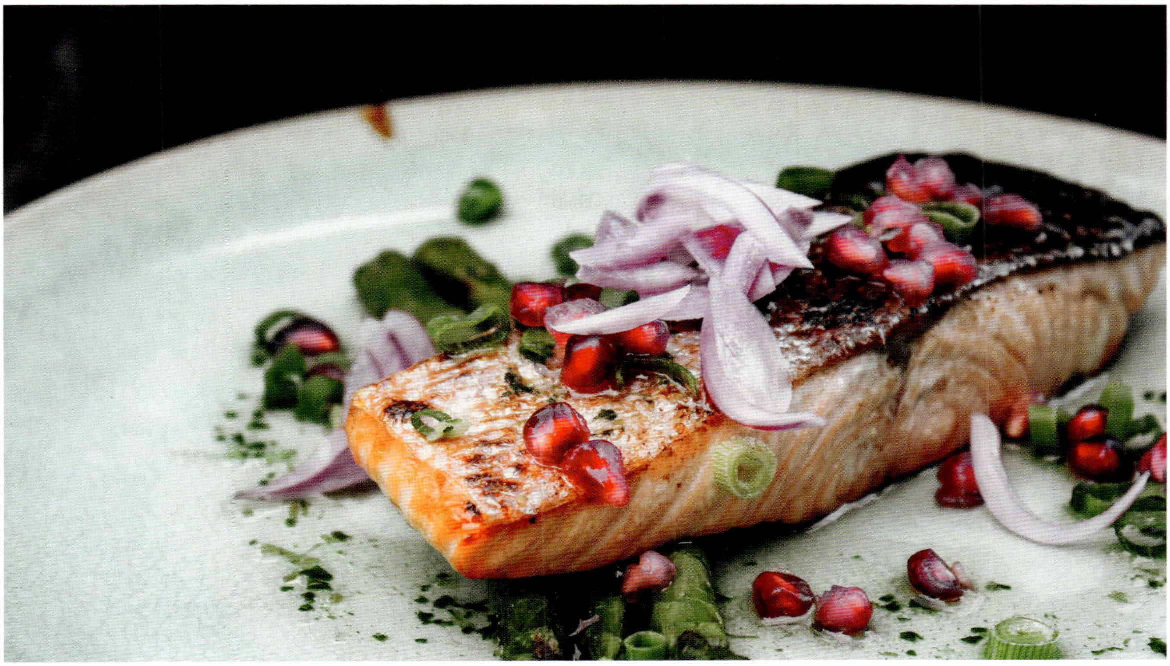

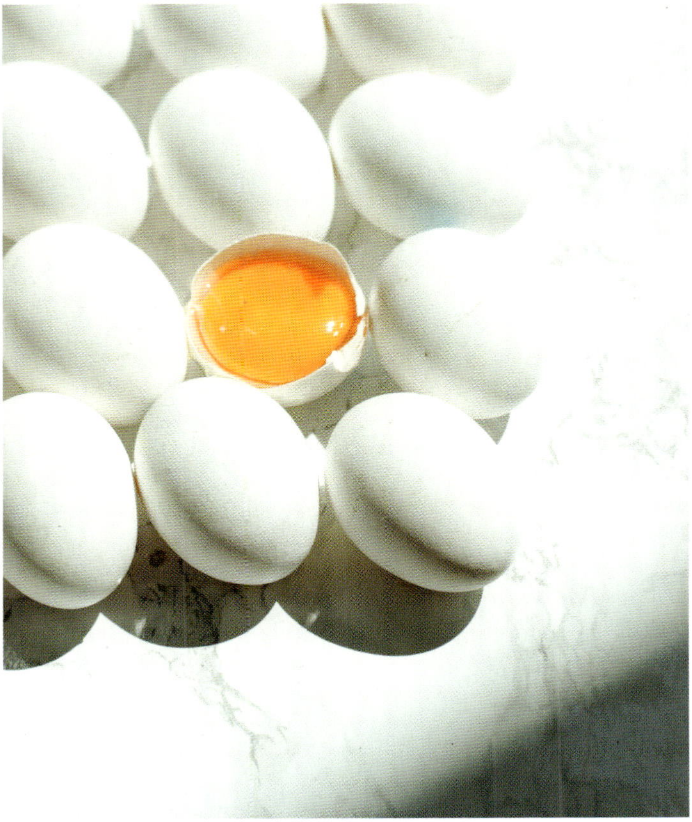

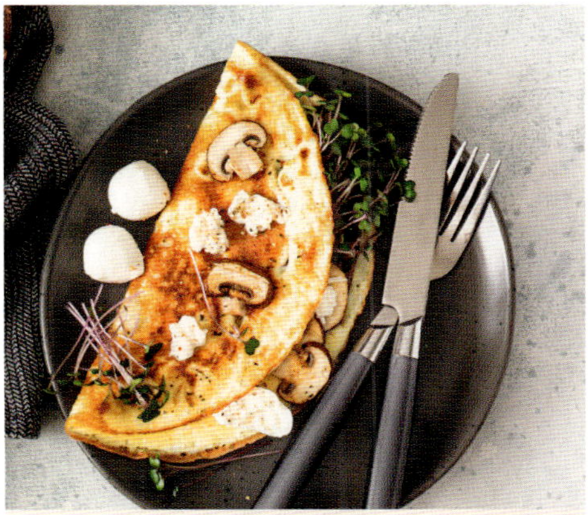

IN THE KITCHEN

EGGS FOR BREAKFAST

Make your breakfast with vitamin D in mind. Cook a three-egg omelet with mushrooms and serve with a small glass of fortified orange juice.

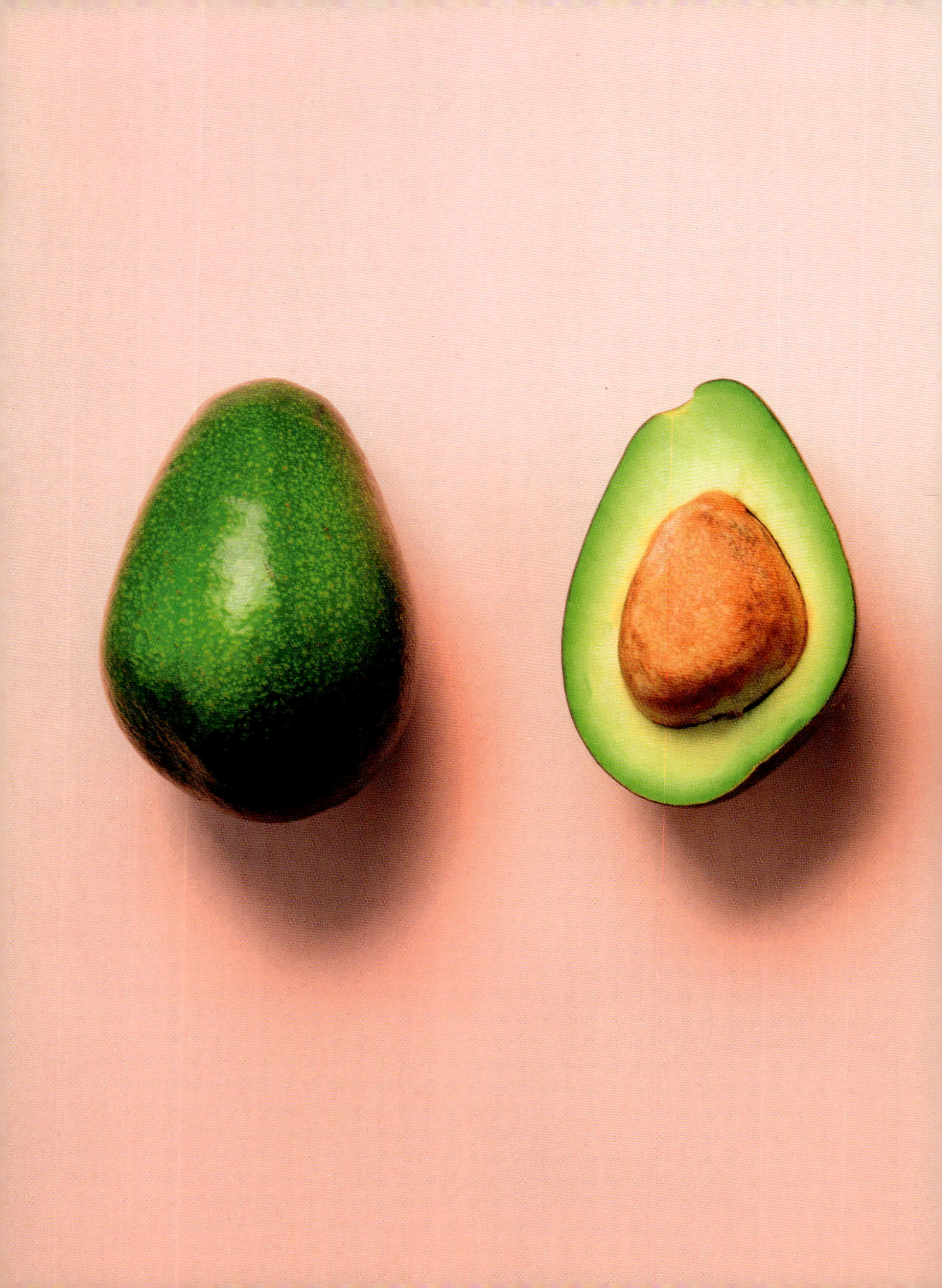

[VITAMIN E]

- TOCOPHEROLS -

THE CELL PROTECTOR

RECOMMENDED DIETARY ALLOWANCE (RDA)

Men and women	15 mg
Pregnancy	15 mg
Lactation	19 mg

"E is for eight" is an easy way to remember some fun facts about fat-soluble vitamin E. This nutrient actually includes eight different chemical forms, but only one form, alpha-tocopherol, is preferred by the human body.

ALL ABOUT TOCOPHEROLS

Vitamin E compounds are well known for their roles as antioxidants, which protect the body's cells from oxidative damage caused by free radicals. This underlying damage in the body may contribute to the development of cancers, heart disease, and other chronic diseases. Exposure to free radicals from UV rays and air pollution can also damage skin cells, and antioxidants such as vitamin E may therefore protect the skin. However, current scientific studies have not found that supplemental vitamin E has significant preventative effects when it comes to disease and skin damage. Getting enough vitamin E from food sources seems to be the best way to meet your needs.

COMMON FOOD SOURCES

Nuts, seeds, and vegetable oils are good sources of vitamin E. To meet the RDA, eat a couple ounces of nuts or seeds several days a week and use olive oil for cooking and in salad dressings.

Sunflower seeds (1 oz, roasted)	7.4 mg
Almonds (1 oz, roasted)	6.8 mg
Wheat germ (1/4 cup)	4.5 mg
Hazelnuts (1 oz, roasted)	4.3 mg
Olive oil (2 tbsp)	4 mg
Dried mango (1 cup)	4 mg
Swiss chard (1 cup, boiled)	3.2 mg
Avocado (1 cup, cubed)	3 mg
Canola oil (1 tbsp)	2.4 mg
Rainbow trout (3 oz, cooked)	2.4 mg
Blackberries (1/2 cup, raw)	0.8 mg

USING SUPPLEMENTS

Vitamin E supplements are rarely necessary, and high doses can cause hemorrhages and strokes. The UL is 1,000 mg per day for adults, but some studies suggest that even lower dosages may increase mortality risk. Individuals taking blood thinners should avoid vitamin E supplements completely.

ROLE IN THE BODY

The main functions of vitamin E are related to its antioxidant capabilities. By intercepting free radicals, vitamin E protects cell membranes and also prevents oxidative damage to low-density lipoproteins (LDLs). This may have benefits for heart health, since oxidized LDLs are thought to contribute to cardiovascular disease.

Furthermore, some observational studies suggest an inverse relationship between vitamin E consumption and the risk of death from heart disease. It's important to note, however, that results of studies have been mixed and almost no clinical studies have found that vitamin E supplementation has heart health benefits, but more research is needed. Vitamin E may also boost immune function, specifically the type of immune response that declines with age.

NOTES ON DEFICIENCY

Vitamin E deficiency is rare, but it has been observed in premature infants, individuals with severe malnutrition, and those who have fat malabsorption, Crohn's disease, or cystic fibrosis. Symptoms of deficiency include muscle weakness, balance issues, and retina damage. Even though vitamin E is thought to help protect against disease, it is not known whether vitamin E insufficiency contributes to an increased risk of chronic diseases.

Inadequate vitamin E intake from dietary sources may be more common. Some data indicates that the average daily intake of alpha-tocopherol among US adults is 7.2 mg, less than half of the RDA of 15 mg.

Caution for smokers

Smokers may have a higher chance of deficiency compared to nonsmokers, since cigarette smoking may decrease blood levels of vitamin E.

DID YOU KNOW?

More than 90% of Americans may not meet the requirements for vitamin E from food sources, but supplements are not the recommended solution.

VIT TIPS

There is some evidence that vitamin E supplements may help reduce symptoms of premenstrual syndrome and pain associated with periods. If you are interested in using vitamin E pills for these issues, discuss with your health care provider first.

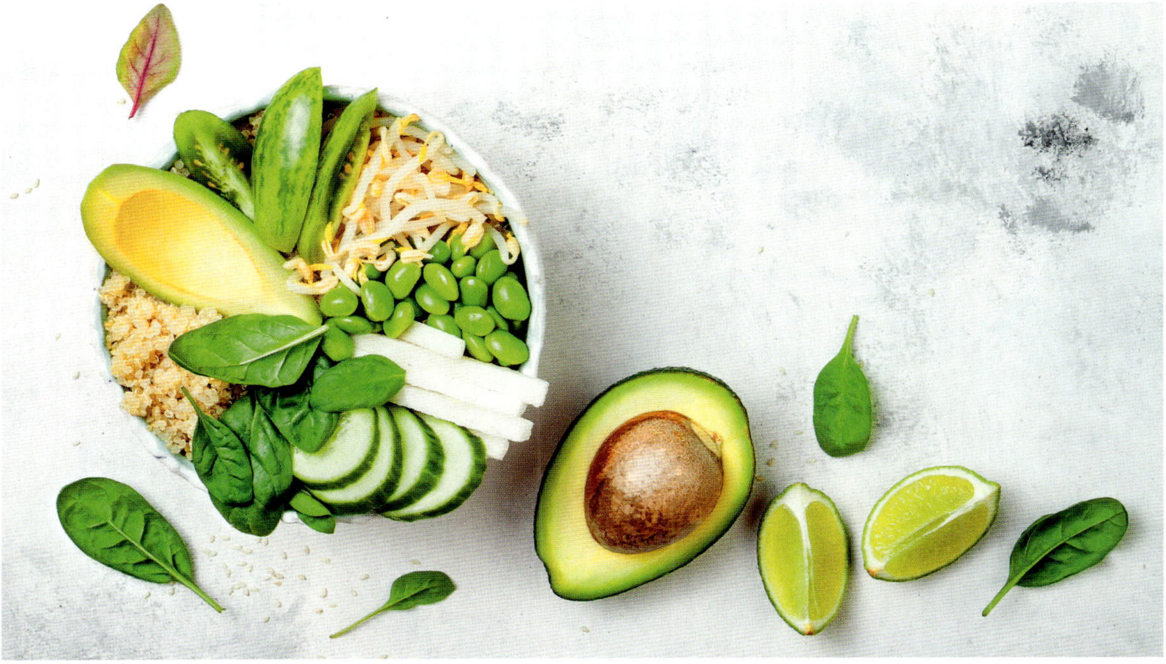

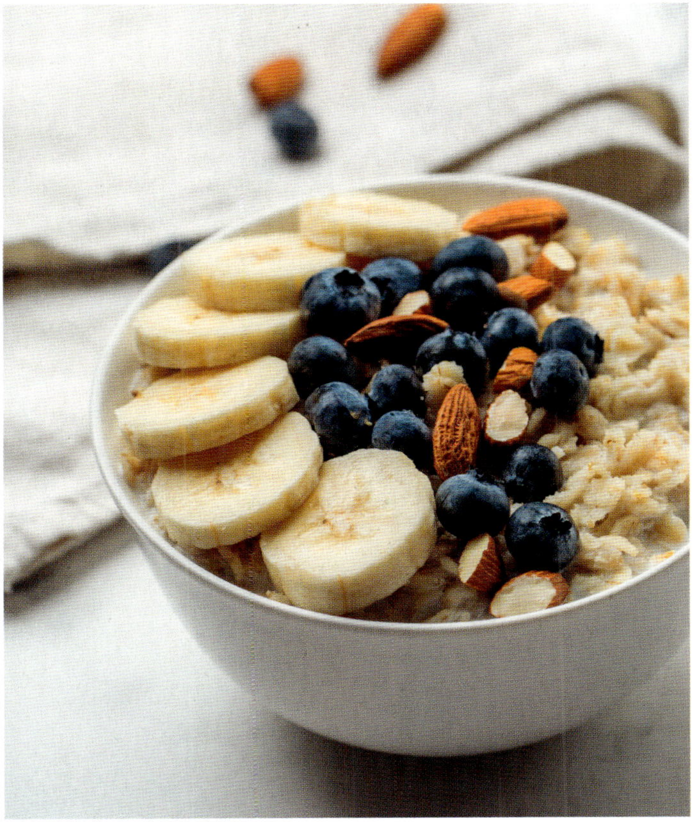

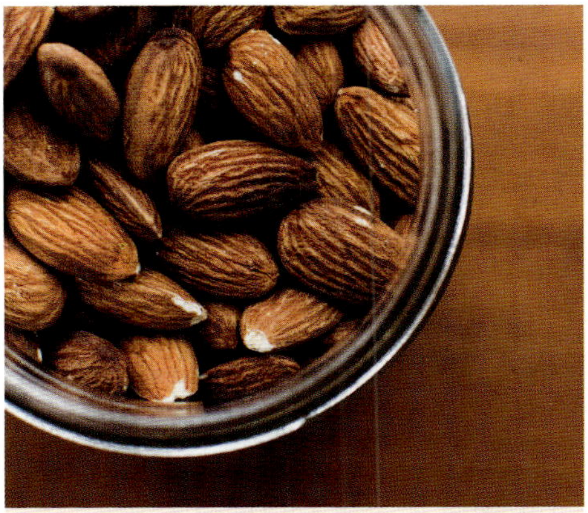

IN THE KITCHEN
NUTTY TRAIL MIX

For a fun snack that's also rich in vitamin E, combine 1/4 cup roasted almonds, 1/4 cup roasted sunflower seeds, 1/4 cup hazelnuts, and 1 cup diced dried mango into a trail mix. This should yield about five servings.

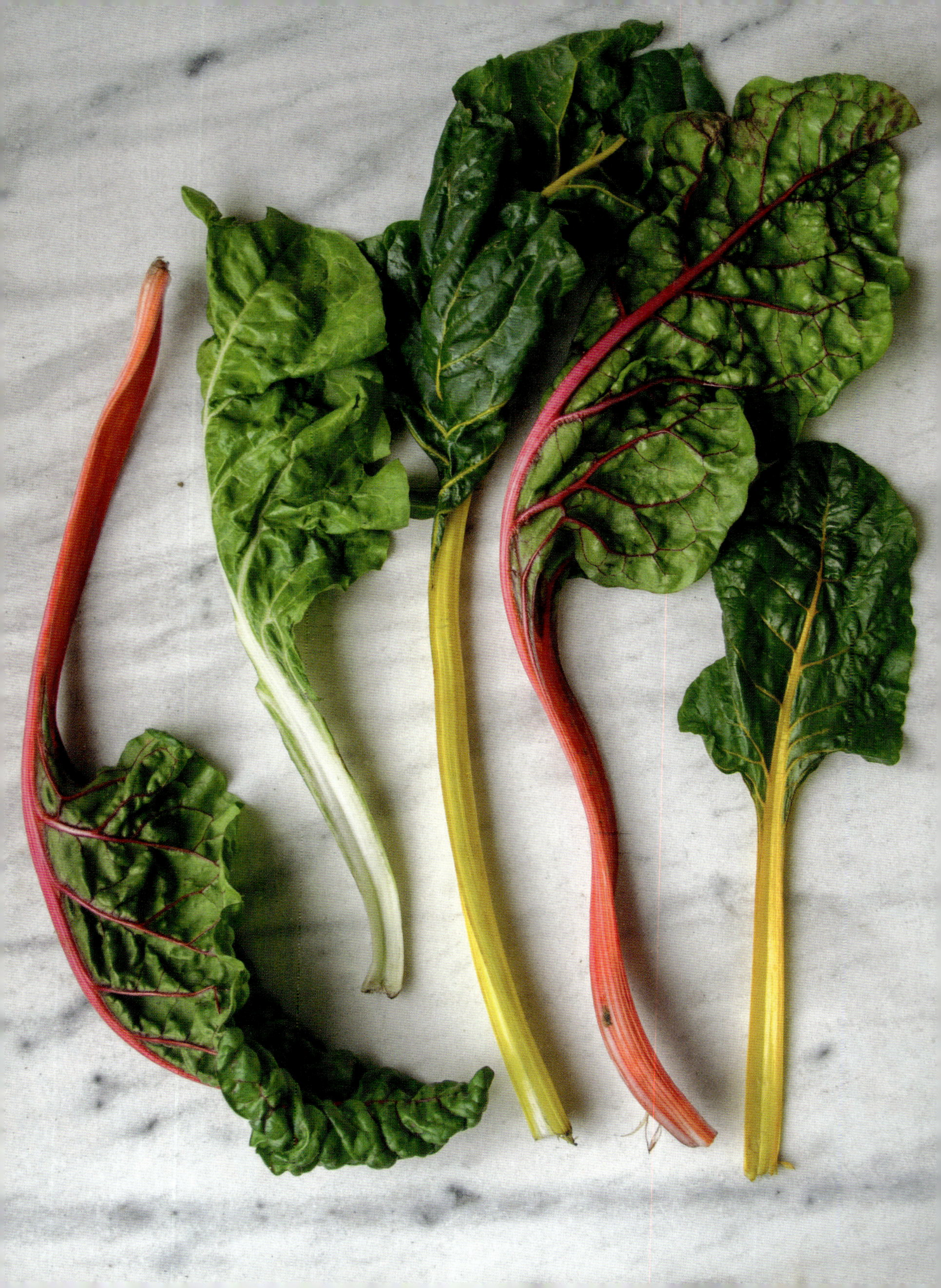

[VITAMIN K]

THE **BLOOD-CLOTTING** VITAMIN

ADEQUATE INTAKE (AI)

Men	120 mcg
Women	90 mcg
Pregnancy and lactation (14–18 years)	75 mcg
Pregnancy and lactation (19+ years)	90 mcg

Did you know that vitamin K got its name from the Danish word "koagulation"? That's because this fat-soluble vitamin is required for proper blood clotting, also known as coagulation.

THE QUINONE FACTOR

Vitamin K refers to a family of compounds that share a common chemical structure, including phylloquinone (vitamin K1) and menaquinones (vitamin K2). Vitamin K1 is the main type found in foods, such as green leafy vegetables, while vitamin K2 is present in some animal products and also synthesized by human gut bacteria.

Most adults get enough vitamin K from their diets, and deficiency in this nutrient is very rare. However, individuals on blood-thinning medications, such as Coumadin (Warfarin), should be aware of their vitamin K consumptions. People who take these medications are advised to maintain a consistent vitamin K intake from foods, so that the drug remains effective.

COMMON FOOD SOURCES

Leafy greens are the best source of vitamin K1; meats, cheese, and other animal products provide vitamin K2, as do some fermented foods, such as natto (fermented soybeans). You can meet your vitamin K needs by eating a few large handfuls of kale or chard a couple days a week, seasoning a few meals with parsley, and serving broccoli with dinner.

Natto (3 oz)	850 mcg
Swiss chard (1 cup, raw)	299 mcg
Parsley (1/4 cup, raw)	246 mcg
Kale (1 cup, raw)	113 mcg
Broccoli (1/2 cup, chopped, boiled)	110 mcg
Iceberg lettuce (1 cup, shredded)	17 mcg
Cashew nuts (1 oz, raw)	9.7 mcg
Ground beef (3 oz, broiled)	6 mcg
Cheddar Cheese (1 1/2 oz)	4 mcg

USING SUPPLEMENTS

Vitamin K is rapidly metabolized and excreted from the body. There is no established UL and it is not considered harmful in high doses. Still, supplements are not necessary for healthy adults.

ROLE IN THE BODY

Vitamin K is vital to proper blood clotting and acts as a cofactor for vitamin-K-dependent carboxylase. This enzyme is involved in the production of blood-clotting proteins, such as prothrombin, also known as clotting factor II.

Osteocalcin, the second-most abundant protein in bones, is another vitamin-K-dependent protein. While the functions of osteocalcin are unclear, it likely plays an important role in bone mineralization and skeletal development. As a result, vitamin K has been the focus of observational studies that suggest higher vitamin K1 intakes are associated with a lower incidence of bone fractures. Still, more research is needed to fully understand the role of vitamin K in bone health.

Vitamin K may also play a role in the prevention of heart disease by stopping the buildup of calcium in arteries, which can contribute to atherosclerosis (a buildup of fatty deposits) and obstruct blood flow.

NOTES ON DEFICIENCY

Vitamin K deficiency is very rare but may occur in individuals with fat malabsorption disorders, cystic fibrosis, celiac disease, or inflammatory bowel disease. In serious cases, it is marked by bleeding and hemorrhage.

Caution for newborns

Newborn babies may also be at risk of deficiency, which can lead to early vitamin K deficiency bleeding (VKDB) in the first week of life or late VKDB in weeks two through twelve. VKDB can cause bleeding in the skin, nose, or even within the skull. To prevent this condition, all babies should be given a dose of vitamin K1 at birth.

DID YOU KNOW?

It took more than 40 years for scientists to determine the role of vitamin K in the body after its initial discovery.

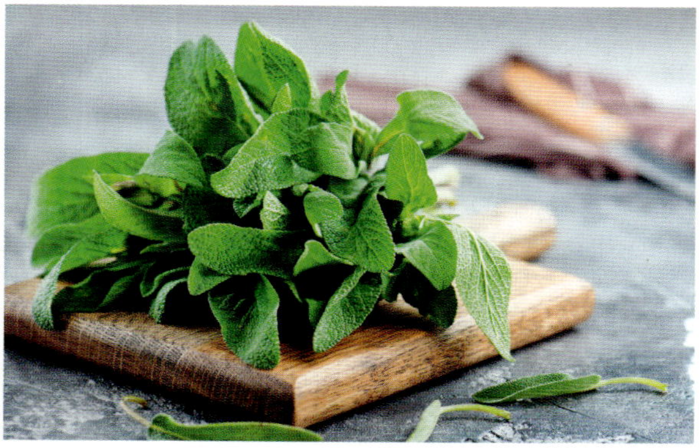

VIT TIPS

Did you know that some herbs and spices are rich in vitamins? One tablespoon of dried sage has 34 mcg of vitamin K—close to 38% of the RDA for women.

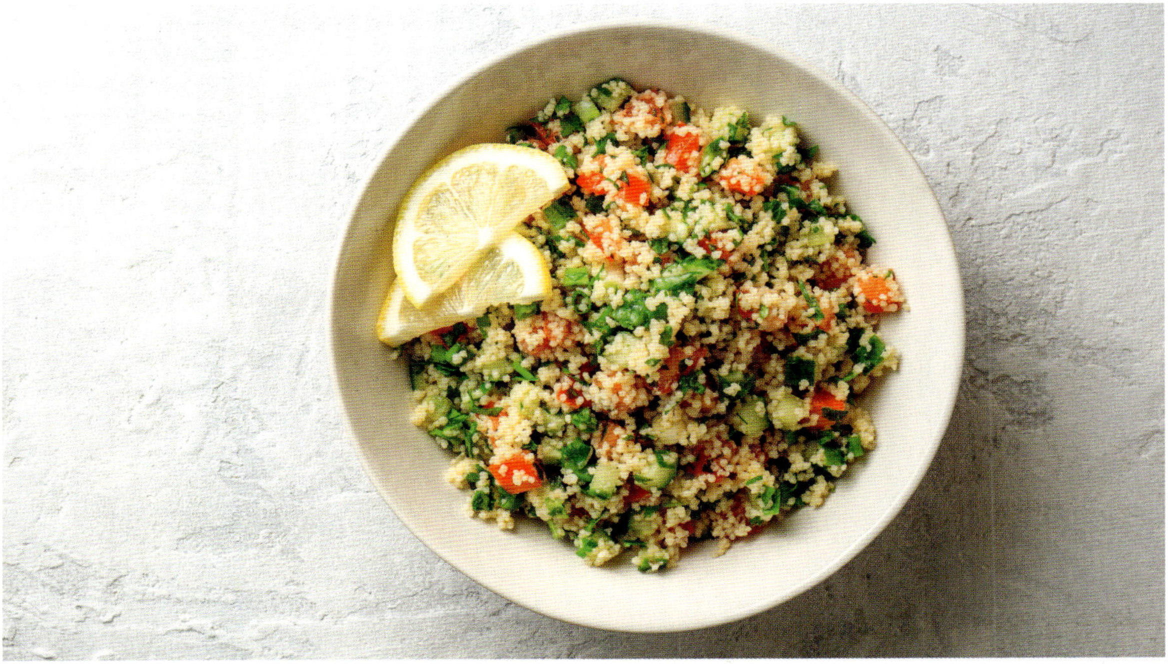

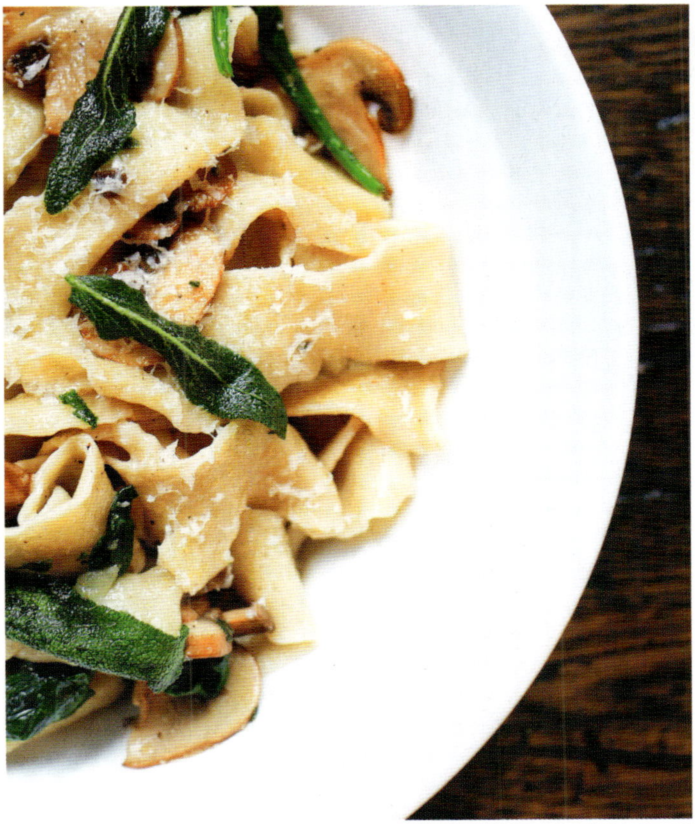

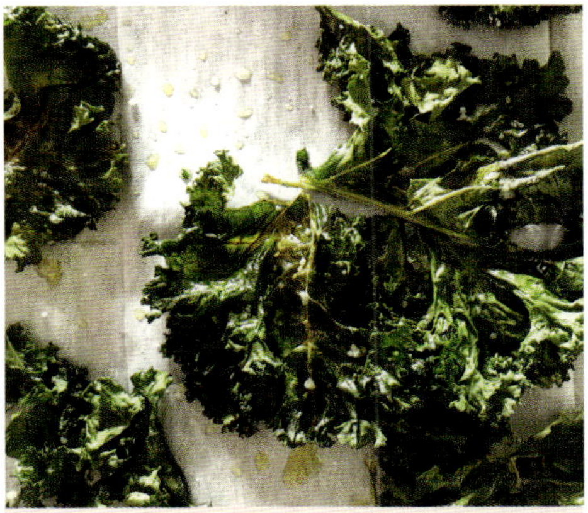

IN THE KITCHEN

CRISPY KALE CHIPS

Remove the stems from a bunch of kale leaves and tear the leaves into smaller pieces. Pat dry and drizzle with 1 tbsp olive oil. Toss, then lay in a single layer on two baking sheets prepared with parchment paper. Season and bake for 25 minutes at 300°F, rotating the baking sheets after 10 minutes.

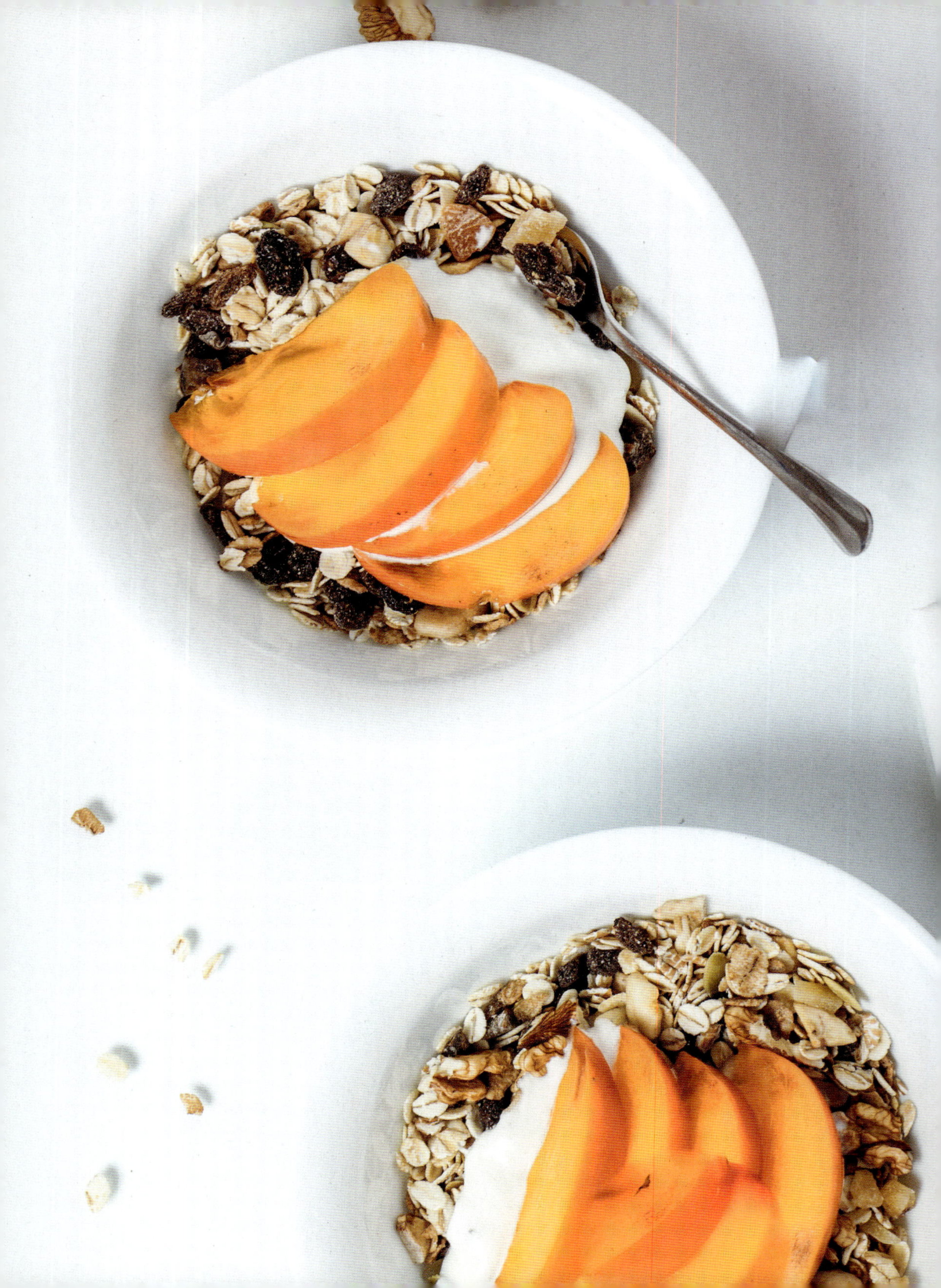

[VITAMIN B1]

- THIAMIN -

RECOMMENDED DIETARY ALLOWANCE (RDA)

Men	1.2 mg
Women	1.1 mg
Pregnancy and lactation	1.4 mg

- THE **FIRST** B VITAMIN -

Ever wonder how B vitamins got their numbers? In the case of thiamin, it's because it was the first B vitamin to be identified.

ALL ABOUT THIAMIN

Discovered in the 1930s, thiamin is a water-soluble vitamin that's essential for energy metabolism in the body. The main active type of thiamin is thiamin diphosphate (TDP), also known as thiamin pyrophosphate (TPP), but it exists in many other forms. When thiamin is consumed from foods, the body converts it to free thiamin so that it can be absorbed. Since thiamin has a short half-life, it's necessary to consume this vitamin frequently from foods. Fortunately, thiamin-rich foods are abundant and commonly consumed in the United States.

USING SUPPLEMENTS

Unless you're at risk of deficiency, taking thiamin supplements is not usually recommended. However, there is no UL for thiamin and no adverse effects have been observed with doses of up to 200 mg per day.

COMMON FOOD SOURCES

Thiamin is added to many cereal and bread products and is naturally present in some meats and fish. About 50% of thiamin intake comes from foods that naturally contain it, such as pork, while the other half comes from fortified and enriched foods. Heating foods, through cooking and pasteurization, decreases thiamin content. You can meet your daily needs by enjoying oatmeal for breakfast and adding beans to lunch or dinner.

Pork chop (5.5 oz, broiled)	0.5 mg
Oats (1 cup, raw)	0.4 mg
Black beans (1/2 cup, boiled)	0.4 mg
Lentils (1 cup, cooked)	0.3 mg
White rice (1 cup, long-grain, enriched, cooked)	0.3 mg
Green peas (1/2 cup, boiled)	0.21 mg
Acorn squash (1/2 cup, cubed, baked)	0.2 mg
Whole wheat bread (1 slice)	0.1 mg
Tuna fish (1 cup, canned in water, drained)	0.06 mg

ROLE IN THE BODY

Thiamin's main function is helping to convert carbohydrates, proteins, and fats from food into usable energy. Specifically, TDP assists enzymes that regulate the metabolism of glucose, amino acids, and fatty acids. Recent research indicates that thiamin may also be a component of brain cell membranes and play a role in brain processes to some extent.

In addition, a small number of studies suggest that adequate thiamin intake may help with blood sugar management in diabetes and possibly slow the development of Alzheimer's disease. More extensive research is needed to better understand the role of thiamin in chronic disease development.

DID YOU KNOW?

Chronic, heavy alcohol consumption is one of the leading causes of thiamin deficiency in the United States.

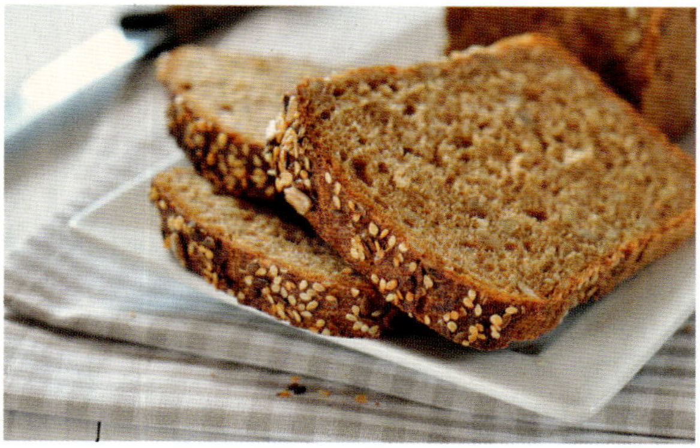

NOTES ON DEFICIENCY

Thiamin deficiency can occur due to insufficient dietary intake, which is rare in the United States. It may also result from reduced absorption, increased needs, and excessive thiamin loss due to illness, medications, or alcohol use.

Beriberi, a disease characterized by wasting, impaired motor functions, and nerve damage in the hands and feet, can result from severe thiamin deficiency. In some instances, beriberi can lead to congestive heart failure.

Caution for heavy drinkers

Since alcohol impairs thiamin absorption, chronic alcohol use can lead to deficiency. Heavy drinkers may also be more likely to eat a poor diet and have inadequate thiamin consumption. Individuals with thiamin deficiency due to alcohol use can develop Wernicke's encephalopathy and eventually Korsakoff's psychosis. These conditions cause abnormal eye movements, balance issues, cognitive impairment, and severe amnesia if left untreated.

VIT VICTORY

The fortification of breads and cereals with thiamin has helped decrease the prevalence of beriberi worldwide.

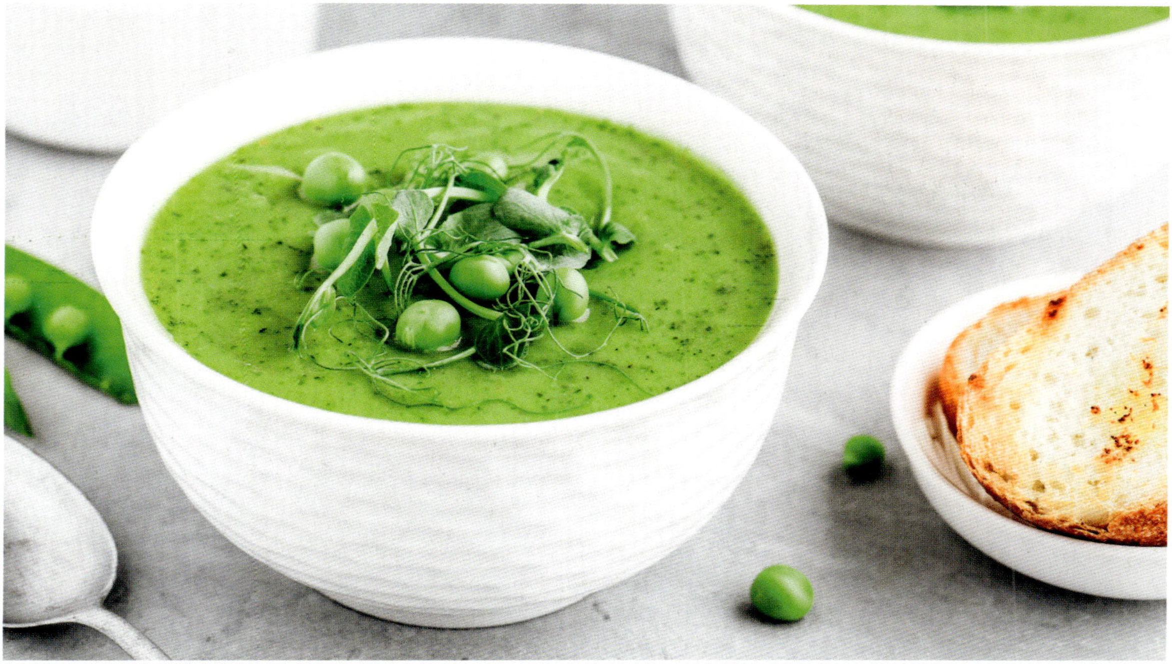

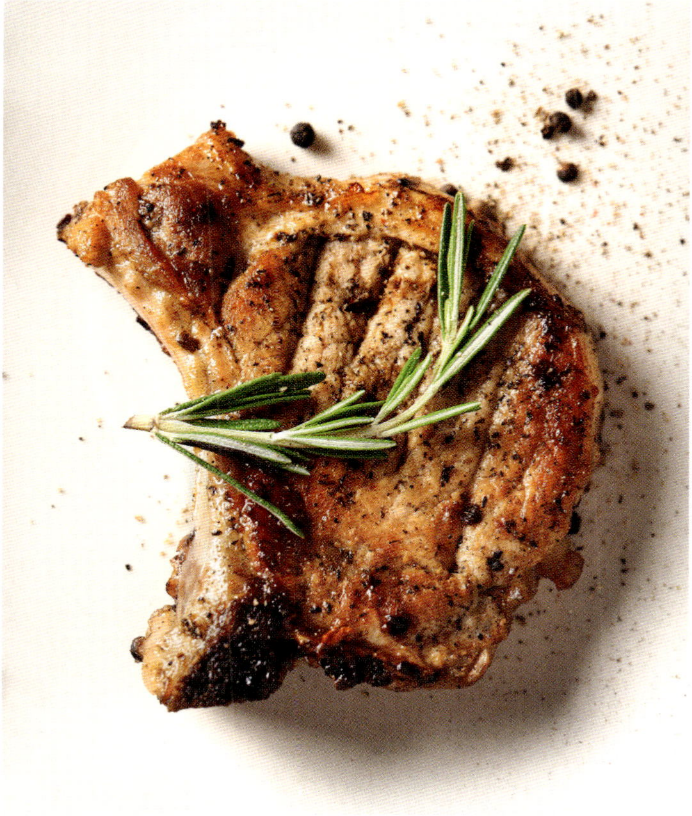

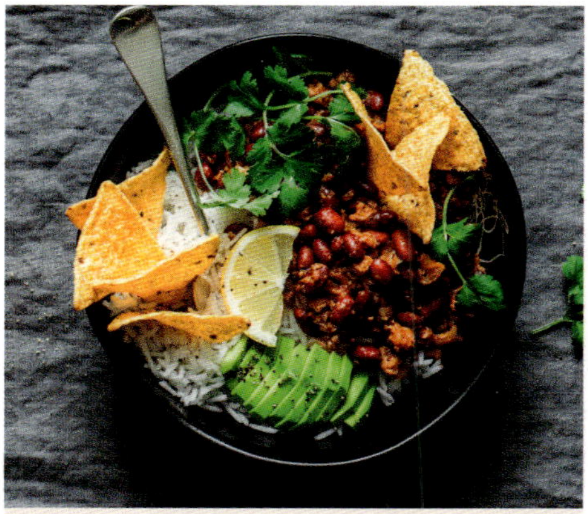

IN THE KITCHEN

B1 BOOSTER

For a thiamin-rich meal, serve baked pork chops with roasted acorn squash or make a burrito bowl with rice and black beans.

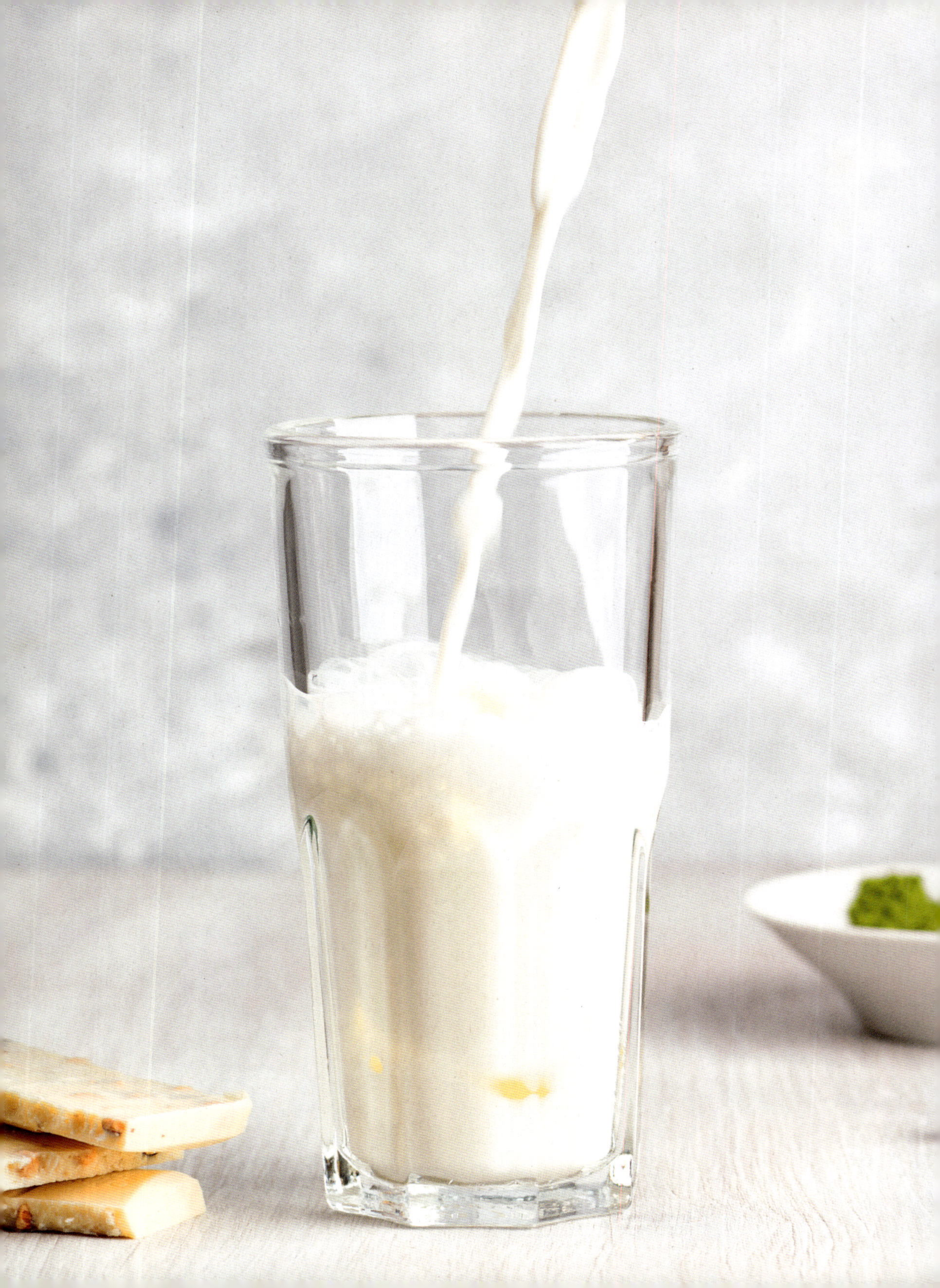

[VITAMIN B2]

- RIBOFLAVIN -

RECOMMENDED DIETARY ALLOWANCE (RDA)

Men	1.3 mg
Women	1.1 mg
Pregnancy	1.4 mg
Lactation	1.6 mg

- THE ENZYME HELPER -

Do you know why milk is no longer stored in glass containers? The answer has to do with riboflavin, also known as vitamin B2.

ALL ABOUT RIBOFLAVIN

Ultraviolet light can deactivate this water-soluble nutrient. So, to preserve the riboflavin in milk, most manufacturers have transitioned to cartons and opaque containers. Milk and dairy products are some of the best sources of riboflavin, but it's found in a variety of veggies, fruits, and fortified cereals and grains, too. Intestinal bacteria can also produce riboflavin, depending on how much is consumed in the diet. Interestingly, the bacteria create more riboflavin after vegetable-based meals compared to meat and animal products.

USING SUPPLEMENTS

Multivitamins and B-complex vitamins contain riboflavin. A healthy adult eating a varied diet does not need riboflavin supplements. There is no UL set for riboflavin, and excess intake of this vitamin from food or supplements is typically excreted in the urine.

COMMON FOOD SOURCES

Riboflavin exists in a few different forms, and more than 90% of dietary riboflavin is flavin mononucleotide (FMN) or flavin adenine dinucleotide (FAD). Both forms are bioavailable and easily absorbed by humans. An adult who eats one cup of yogurt or a couple eggs for breakfast could meet the rest of their daily riboflavin needs by snacking on a handful of almonds.

Oatmeal (1 cup, fortified, cooked with water)	1.1 mg
Plain yogurt (1 cup, nonfat)	0.6 mg
2% milk (1 cup)	0.5 mg
Beef steak (4 oz, braised)	0.32 mg
Almonds (1 oz, roasted)	0.3 mg
Egg (1 large, hard-boiled)	0.26 mg
Quinoa (1 cup, cooked)	0.2 mg
Asparagus (8 spears, boiled)	0.17 mg
Chicken (3 oz, dark meat, roasted)	0.16 mg

ROLE IN THE BODY

As a major component of the coenzymes FMN and FAD, riboflavin is vital for processes related to energy production, metabolism, and cellular function in the body. In particular, FAD assists with the electron transport chain, a key aspect of energy production.

Riboflavin-dependent enzymes also play a role in the body's antioxidant defenses. Glutathione reductase, for example, is an enzyme that requires FAD and protects cells from free radicals and oxidative damage.

Some evidence points to riboflavin's possible role in the treatment of migraine headaches. A handful of randomized, controlled trials have found that supplemental riboflavin may help reduce the frequency of migraines when used with pharmacological interventions.

DID YOU KNOW?

About two times as much riboflavin is lost when foods are boiled, compared to techniques that do not use as much cooking water.

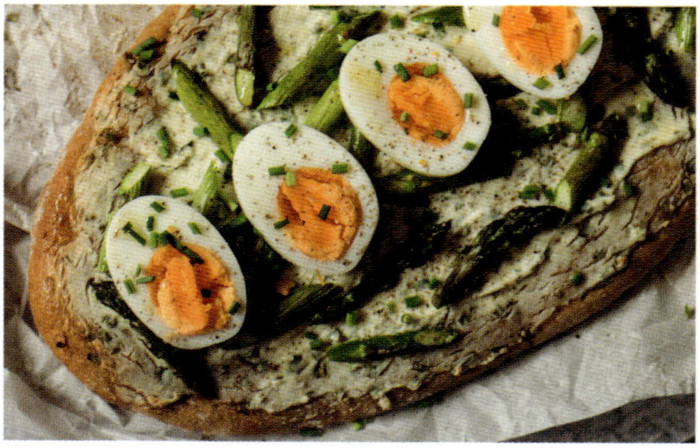

NOTES ON DEFICIENCY

Riboflavin deficiency is a very rare issue in the United States. However, some population groups may not get enough riboflavin if they don't consume meat or dairy products.

Caution for vegetarian and vegan athletes

Vegetarian and vegan athletes may be at greater risk of inadequate riboflavin consumption, since intense exercise puts stress on the energy pathways in the body that use riboflavin.

Caution in pregnancy

Pregnant women should make sure to consume enough riboflavin-rich foods, since some research suggests that riboflavin deficiency can increase the risk of high blood pressure during pregnancy and lead to poor birth outcomes for infants.

What are the symptoms?

Signs of riboflavin deficiency include angular stomatitis, which is marked by lesions that develop at the corners of the mouth, and cheilosis, marked by swollen and cracked lips. At-risk groups can increase riboflavin consumption by eating more fortified whole grains, almonds, spinach, and asparagus if they choose to avoid animal products.

VIT TIPS

To preserve the riboflavin content of asparagus, try steaming, microwaving, sautéing, or pan-frying instead of boiling or roasting.

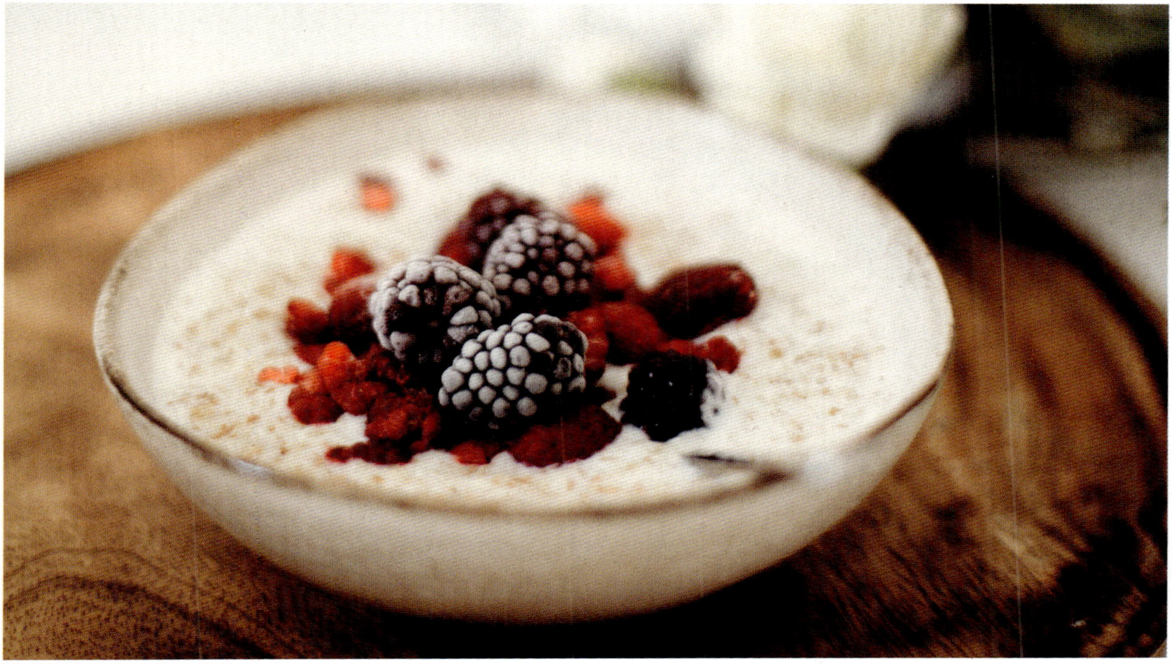

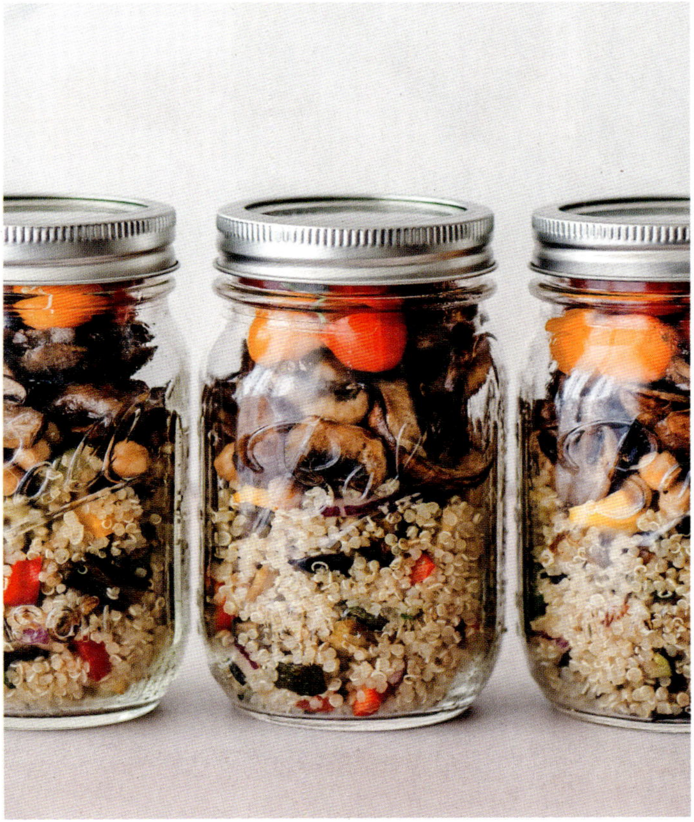

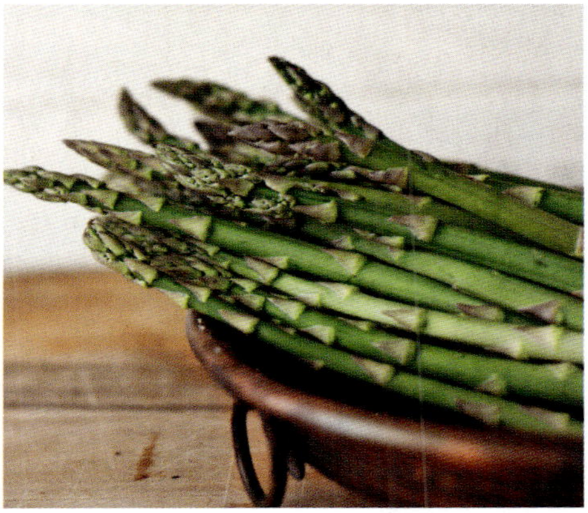

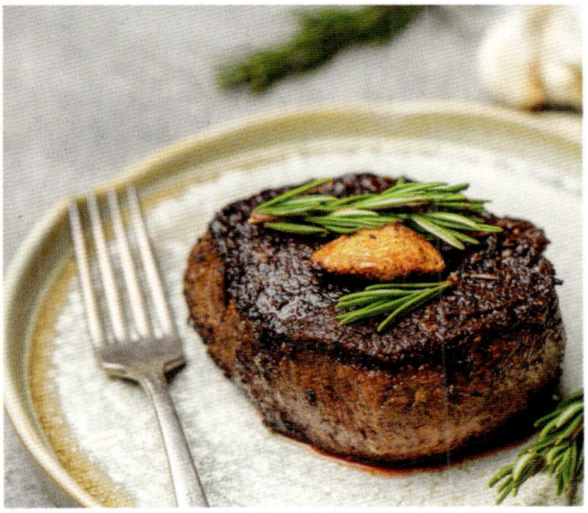

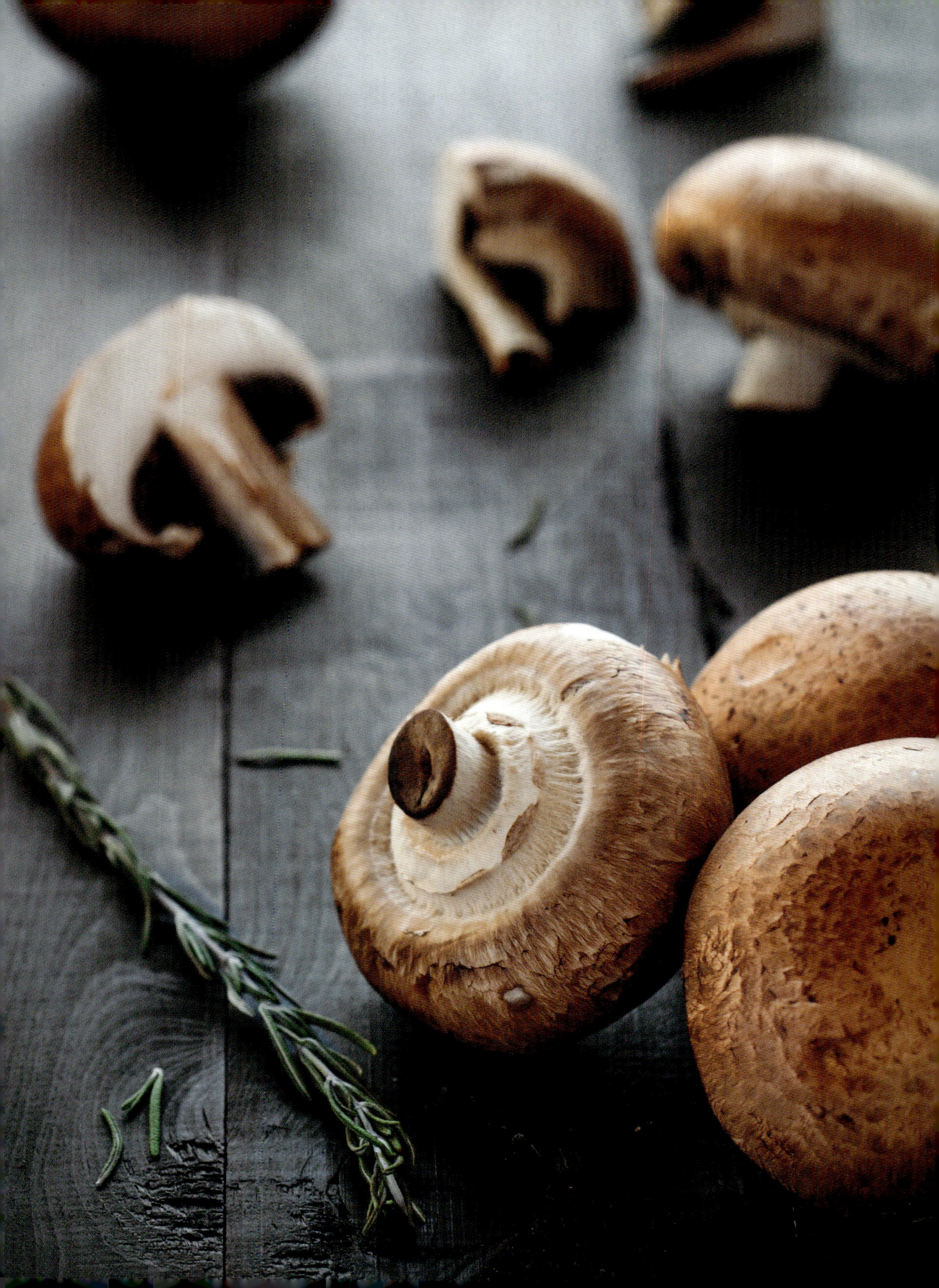

[VITAMIN B3]

- NIACIN -

THE DNA REPAIRER

RECOMMENDED DIETARY ALLOWANCE (RDA)

Men	16 mg NE
Women	14 mg NE
Pregnancy	18 mg NE
Lactation	17 mg NE

NE: niacin equivalents

Niacin may seem like just another water-soluble B vitamin, but it's required for more than 400 enzymes in the body!

ALL ABOUT NIACIN

The name niacin refers to a group of compounds found in foods and supplements, which are then converted into the coenzyme nicotinamide adenine dinucleotide (NAD) by tissues.

NAD is a metabolically active form of niacin, and it can also be further converted into another active coenzyme known as nicotinamide adenine dinucleotide phosphate (NADP). NAD and NADP help with energy production, gene expression, DNA repair, and antioxidant functions.

The RDAs for niacin are listed in niacin equivalents (NE). This is because both niacin, as well as the amino acid tryptophan, which can be converted into NAD by the liver, are considered sources of niacin in the food supply. Most Americans get plenty of niacin from their daily diets.

COMMON FOOD SOURCES

Both animal and plant foods contain niacin. Tryptophan-rich foods that provide NE include turkey, chicken, peanuts, and pumpkin seeds, among others. Eating a variety of proteins, such as chicken, turkey, and salmon throughout the week is an easy way to get enough of this vitamin.

Chicken breast (3 oz, grilled)	10.3 mg
Turkey breast (3 oz, roasted)	10 mg
Sockeye salmon (3 oz, cooked)	8.6 mg
Portabellos (1 cup, grilled)	7.6 mg
Brown rice (1 cup, cooked)	5.2 mg
Peanuts (1 oz, roasted)	4.2 mg
Russet potato (1 medium, baked)	2.3 mg
Pumpkin seeds (1 oz, roasted)	1.3 mg
Bulgur (1 cup, cooked)	0.9 mg
Raisins (1/4 cup)	0.3 mg

USING SUPPLEMENTS

Niacin exists in many different forms in supplements, including B-complex vitamins. High doses can cause unpleasant skin flushing. Healthy adults do not need supplements, but they may be used in some disease treatments.

ROLE IN THE BODY

As coenzymes, NAD and NADP are primarily involved in electron-transfer reactions, meaning they are necessary for reactions that produce energy from the breakdown of carbs, fats, proteins, and alcohol. NADP, in particular, helps with the creation of fatty acids and cholesterol, as well as components of antioxidants.

The form of niacin known as nicotinic acid may help reduce blood cholesterol levels. It's unclear how exactly nicotinic acid works, but prescription medications with this compound are sometimes used in combination with statins to treat high cholesterol and triglycerides. Nicotinic acid may also increase concentrations of high-density lipoprotein (HDL) cholesterol, which is considered the "good" cholesterol. Finally, NAD is vital for DNA repair in the body, and niacin could therefore be involved in cancer prevention. Some observational studies suggest that nicotinamide, another form of niacin, may help reduce the occurrence of premalignant skin cancer lesions.

NOTES ON DEFICIENCY

Most Americans get more than the RDA for niacin from foods, and so deficiency is rare in the United States. However, people with severe malnutrition or genetic disorders that interfere with tryptophan absorption may be at risk of deficiency.

The disease that results from severe niacin deficiency is known as pellagra, and is marked by a bright red tongue, skin rashes, brown skin discoloration after sun exposure, and digestive issues. Eventually, pellagra can lead to hallucinations, fatigue, apathy, and, in some cases, death.

DID YOU KNOW?

Even though they have similar names, nicotinic acid and nicotinamide are not related to nicotine found in tobacco.

FACT OR FICTION?

While it is true that some nutrients may be more concentrated in the skin of vegetables (and just below the surface) than in the flesh, potatoes with or without skin provide similar amounts of niacin.

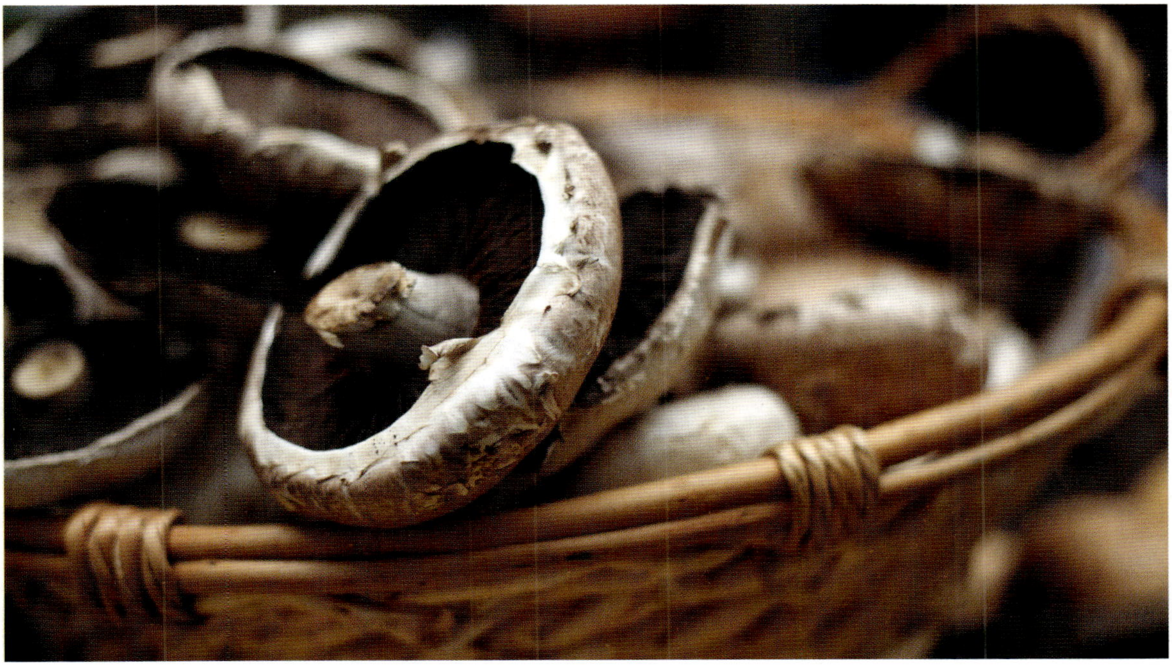

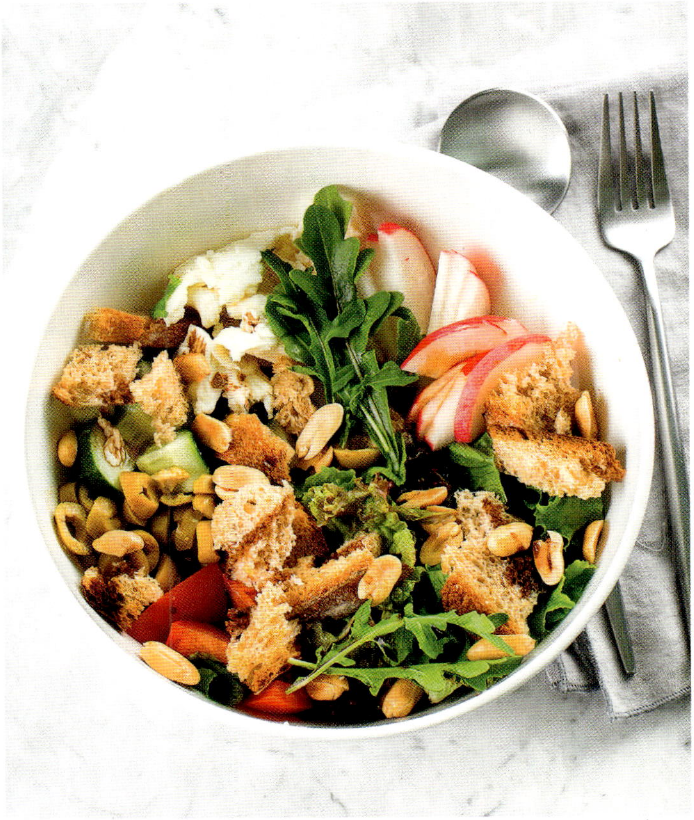

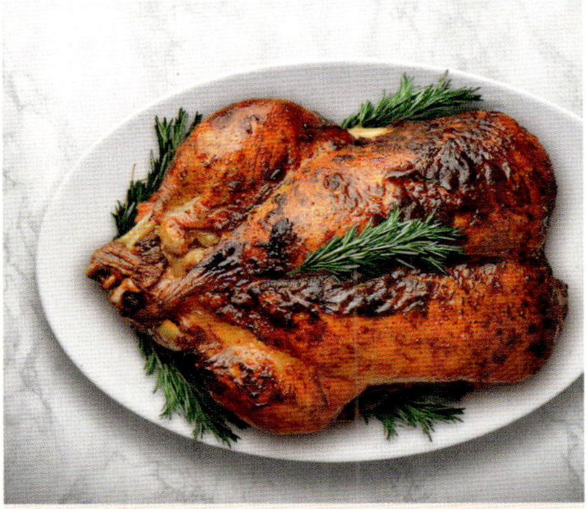

IN THE KITCHEN

ROAST TURKEY SUPPER

To build a healthy meal that's loaded with niacin, serve roasted turkey breast with a baked Russet potato and sautéed portabello mushrooms.

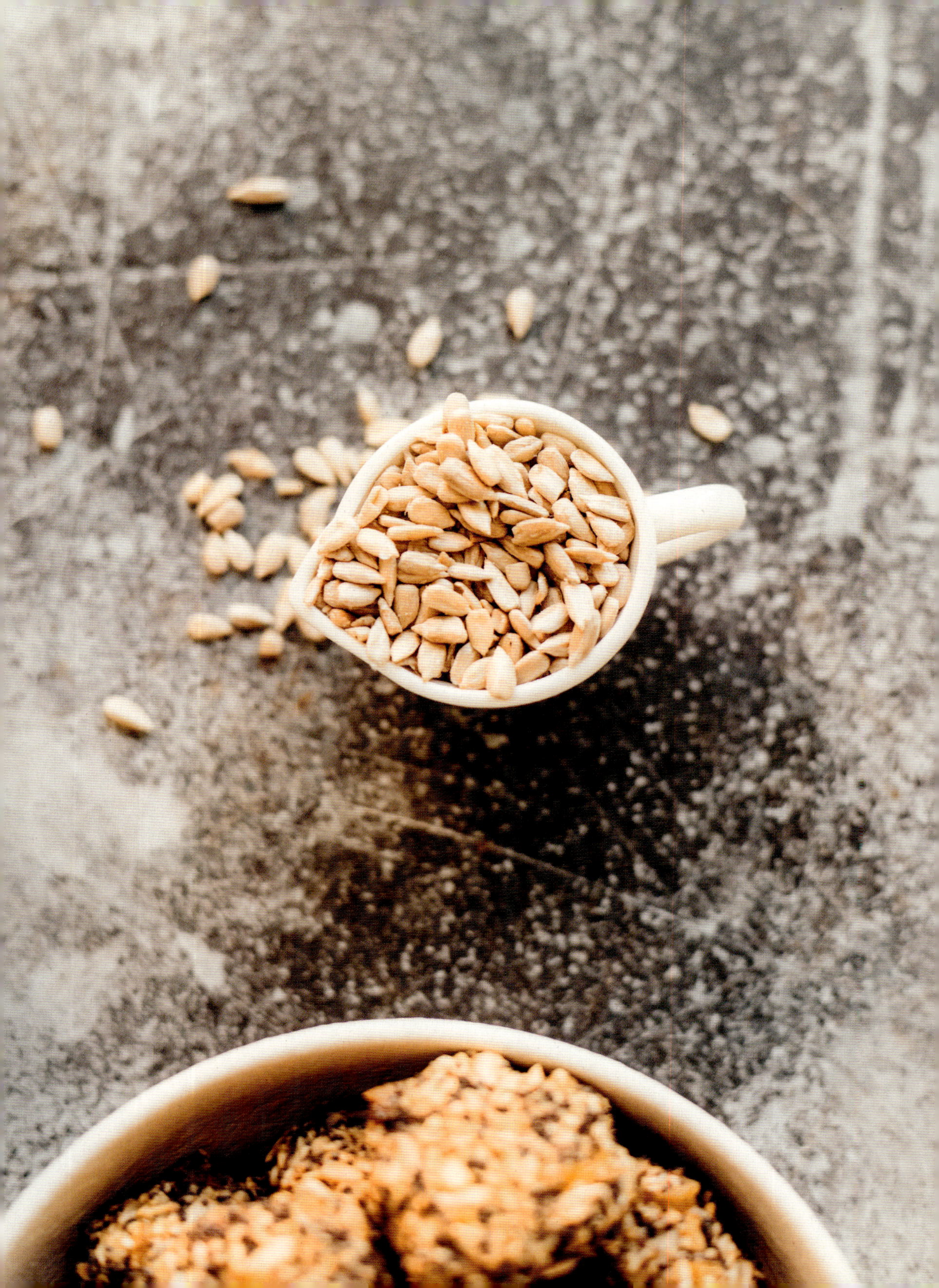

[VITAMIN B5]

- PANTOTHENIC ACID -

ADEQUATE INTAKE (AI)

Men and women	5 mg
Pregnancy	6 mg
Lactation	7 mg

- THE "EVERYWHERE" VITAMIN -

Most nutrients were named for a specific reason, including vitamin B5, also known as pantothenic acid. This name comes from the Greek word pantos, meaning "everywhere," highlighting the abundance of this vitamin in the food supply.

ALL ABOUT PANTOTHENIC ACID

Pantothenic acid is a water-soluble nutrient that assists in a number of essential functions in the body. It's necessary for the creation of coenzyme A (CoA), which takes part in processes that turn food into usable energy.

Since pantothenic acid is so widely available in the diet, deficiency of this vitamin is very rare today. However, history tells a different story. Malnourished World War II prisoners in the Philippines and Japan reportedly experienced symptoms of pantothenic acid deficiency, such as burning, tingling, and numbness in their feet. These symptoms resolved after supplementation with vitamin B5, giving scientists insight into what happens with deficiency of this specific nutrient.

COMMON FOOD SOURCES

Similar to other B vitamins, pantothenic acid exists in both animal and plant foods. Breakfast cereals and other foods may also be fortified with pantothenic acid. Just ½ cup of sunflower seeds provides enough pantothenic acid for your daily needs. Incorporating avocado, sweet potato, broccoli, chicken, and eggs on a weekly basis is another good way to meet your needs.

Beef liver (3 oz, cooked)	5.6 mg
Sunflower seeds (¼ cup, raw)	2.4 mg
Chicken breast (3 oz, roasted)	1.3 mg
Avocado (½ fruit, sliced)	1 mg
Sweet potato (½ cup, cooked with skin)	1 mg
2% milk (1 cup)	0.9 mg
Egg (1 large, hard-boiled)	0.7 mg
Broccoli (½ cup, boiled)	0.5 mg
Cheddar cheese (1.5 oz)	0.2 mg

USING SUPPLEMENTS

With such an abundance of naturally occurring pantothenic acid in common foods, supplements are not necessary.

ROLE IN THE BODY

The main function of pantothenic acid is to assist in the synthesis of coenzyme A. Derivatives of coenzyme A are necessary for generating energy from the breakdown of fats, carbohydrates, and proteins and creating fatty acids. They also take part in the production of melatonin, the hormone that regulates the sleep-wake cycle.

Pantothenic acid may influence the synthesis of blood lipids, such as triglycerides. For this reason, clinical trials have explored the use of pantethine, a form of pantothenic acid, in therapeutic doses for the reduction of lipid levels. Pantethine supplements have been shown to decrease triglycerides, cholesterol, and "bad" LDL cholesterol, while increasing "good" HDL cholesterol. Improvements in blood lipid levels may decrease the risk of heart disease. Initial research on pantethine appears promising, but more studies are needed to better understand the roles of vitamin B5 in heart health.

NOTES ON DEFICIENCY

Pantothenic acid deficiency is rarely seen, except in cases of severe malnutrition. In most instances, people with a deficiency also have insufficient levels of other nutrients. Therefore, it is difficult to identify the characterizations of true pantothenic acid deficiency. However, based on the information learned from the World War II prisoners who experienced deficiency, signs and symptoms include numbness and burning in the hands and feet, as well as a general restlessness and irritability.

DID YOU KNOW?

The liver needs coenzyme A, derived from vitamin B5, to metabolize several drugs and toxins.

VIT TIPS

It's best to get pantothenic acid from fresh whole food sources that have had minimal processing. This is because food processing can decrease the pantothenic acid content of animal and plant foods by 20–80%.

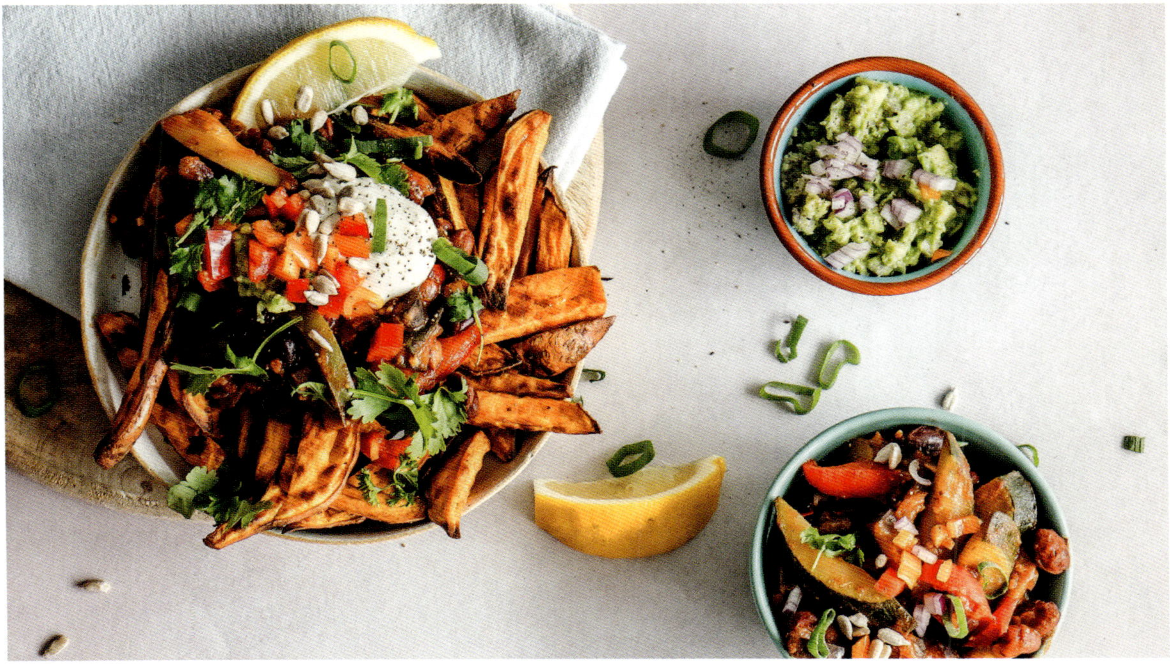

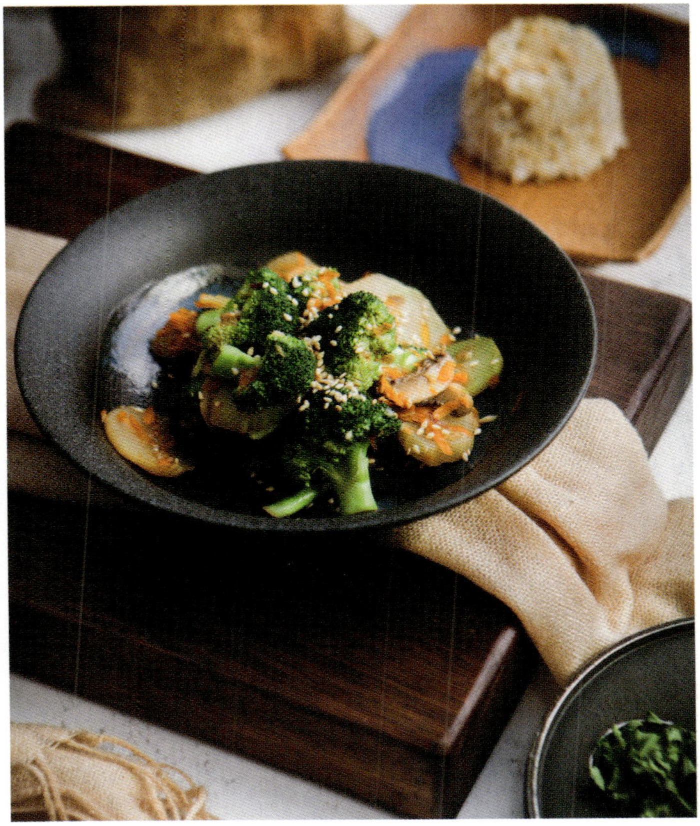

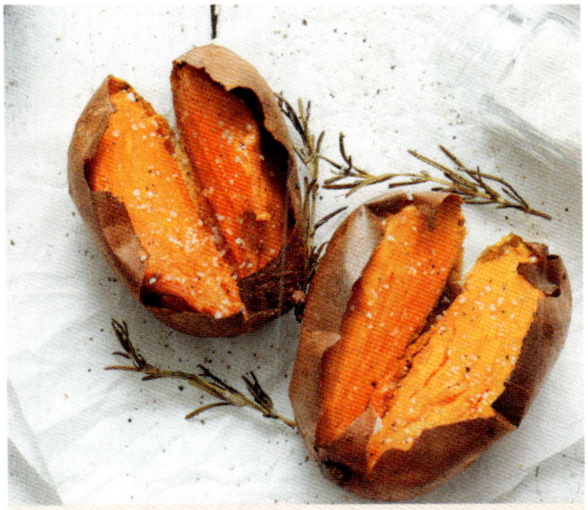

IN THE KITCHEN

SWEET POTATO LUNCH

Baked sweet potatoes topped with avocado and sunflower seeds make a delicious meal high in vitamin B5.

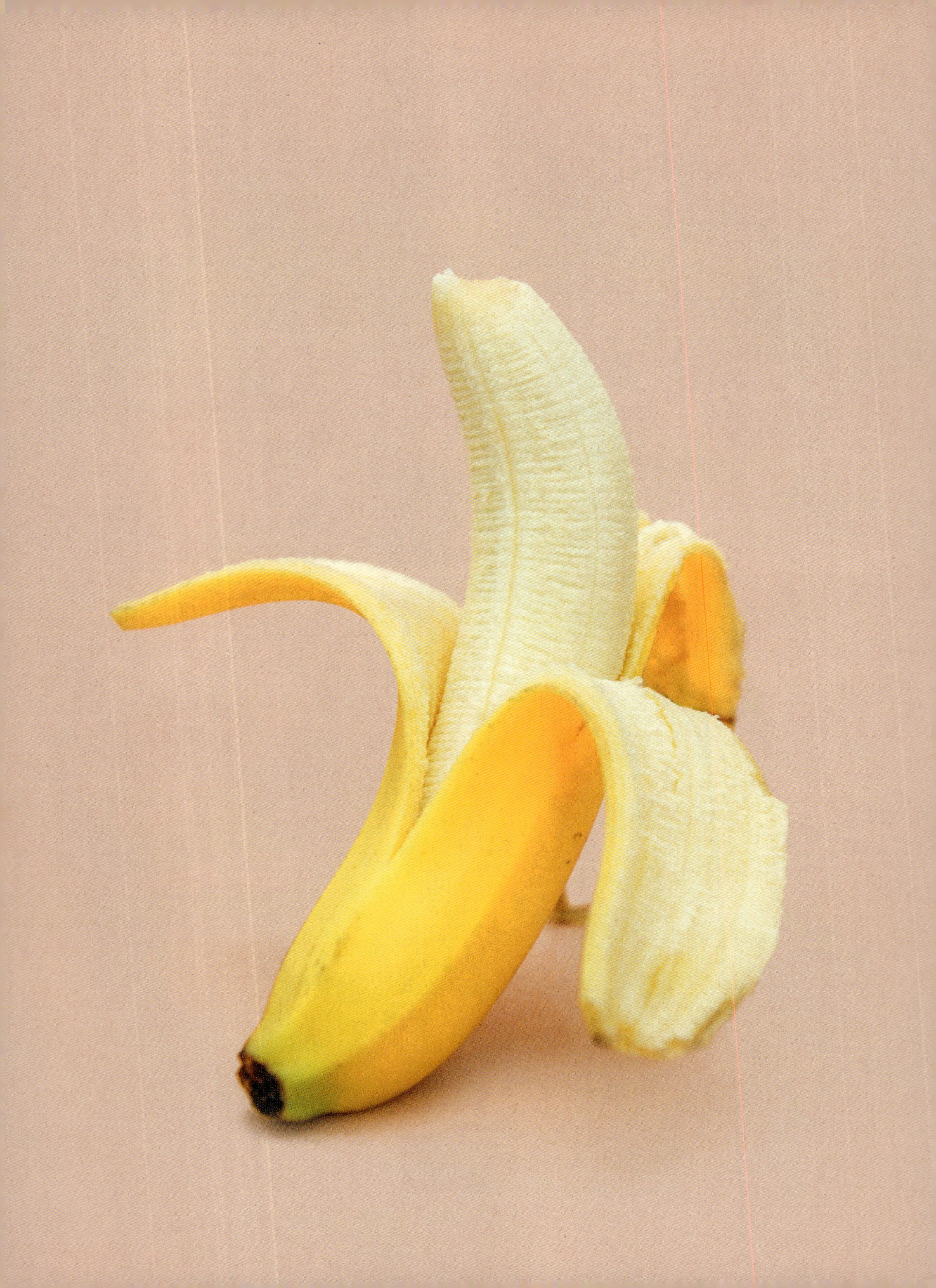

[VITAMIN B6]

– PYRIDOXINE –

THE PROTEIN **CREATOR**

RECOMMENDED DIETARY ALLOWANCE (RDA)

Men and women (19–50 years)	1.3 mg
Men (51+ years)	1.7 mg
Women (51+ years)	1.5 mg
Pregnancy	1.9 mg
Lactation	2 mg

Question: What do heart disease, premenstrual syndrome (PMS), and morning sickness have in common? Answer: Vitamin B6 may be helpful in managing all of them!

ALL ABOUT PYRIDOXINE

This water-soluble nutrient, also known as pyridoxine, refers to a group of six compounds that perform similar activities in the body. The active forms of vitamin B6 are the pyridoxal 5' phosphate (PLP) and pyridoxamine 5' phosphate (PMP). These coenzymes are involved in more than 100 processes in the body, including protein metabolism and the creation of red blood cells.

With so many important functions, it's vital to get enough vitamin B6 from your diet. Fortunately, this is not an issue for the majority of adults in the United States, as B6 is abundant in the food supply.

COMMON FOOD SOURCES

Vitamin B6 is found in meat and fish, but also in beans and fortified cereals. Together, turkey and a baked potato provide enough vitamin B6 to meet the RDA, and just a cup of canned chickpeas has close to 100% of your needs.

Breakfast cereal (1 cup, fortified)	0.5–2.5 mg
Chickpeas (1 cup, canned)	1.1 mg
Wheat bran (1 cup)	0.8 mg
Russet potato (1 medium, baked, with skin)	0.7 mg
Turkey (3 oz, light meat, cooked)	0.6 mg
Sockeye salmon (3 oz, cooked)	0.6 mg
Banana (1 medium)	0.4 mg
Dried plums (1 cup)	0.36 mg
1% cottage cheese (1 cup)	0.2 mg
Hazelnuts (1 oz, roasted)	0.18 mg

USING SUPPLEMENTS

Vitamin B6 can cause pain and numbness in the hands and feet in high supplemental doses. Supplements may be recommended for certain conditions, but should be taken with caution. The UL is set at 100 mg per day for adults.

ROLE IN THE BODY

PLP, one of the coenzymes derived from pyridoxine, is best known for its role in generating energy from amino acids, in the form of glucose. But the functions of PLP don't stop there.

Enzymes dependent on PLP in the brain are responsible for the creation of serotonin and dopamine, two neurotransmitters that regulate mood. PLP also assists with the creation of hemoglobin, the main protein in red blood cells that enables them to transport oxygen in the body. In addition, vitamin B6 may help decrease blood levels of homocysteine, another protein that can increase the risk of heart disease when present in elevated levels in the blood.

There are many other functions of vitamin B6 that have made it a nutrient of interest for the prevention and management of illness. Vitamin B6 supplements have been used since the 1940s to treat morning sickness, and limited evidence suggests that they may also improve symptoms of PMS.

NOTES ON DEFICIENCY

Symptoms of vitamin B6 deficiency, albeit uncommon, include microcytic anemia, swollen tongue, cracks at the corner of the mouth, and weakened immunity. Groups at risk of vitamin B6 deficiency include individuals with end-stage kidney disease or impaired kidney function, rheumatoid arthritis, and Crohn's disease, ulcerative colitis, celiac disease, or another condition that causes nutrient malabsorption.

DID YOU KNOW?

Emerging research suggests that low vitamin B6 levels in the body may be linked to depression, but more studies are needed.

VIT TIPS

B vitamins are water-soluble and can be excreted in the urine, but you can experience negative side effects with high dosages of some supplemental forms. This is not the case with B vitamins that naturally exist in appropriate amounts in foods.

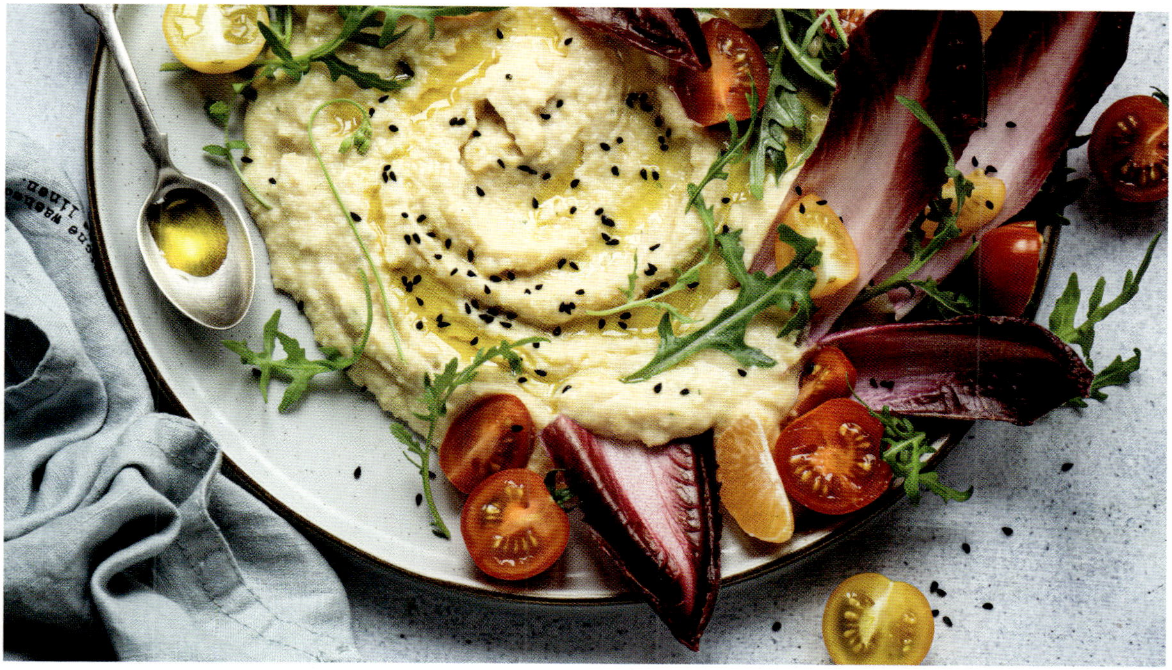

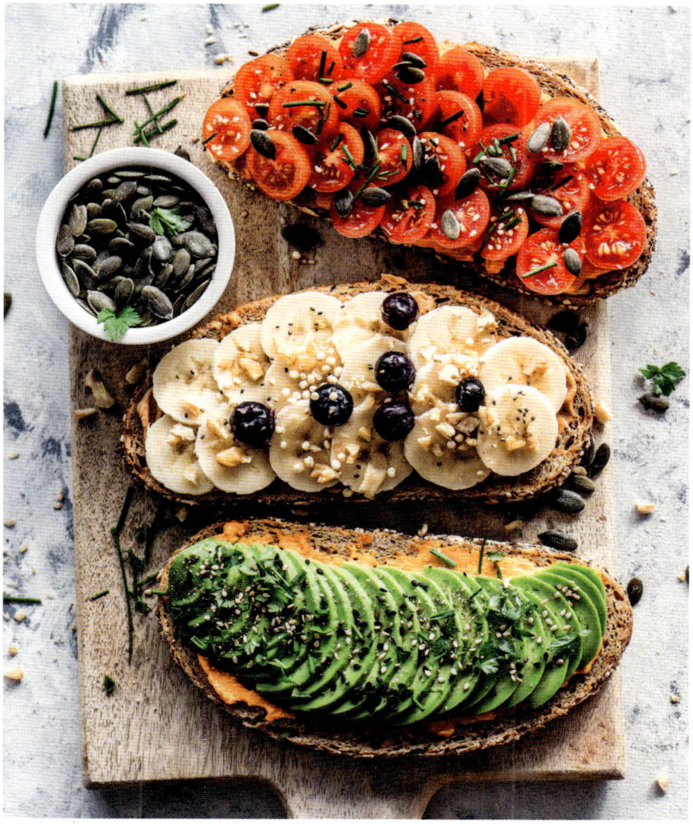

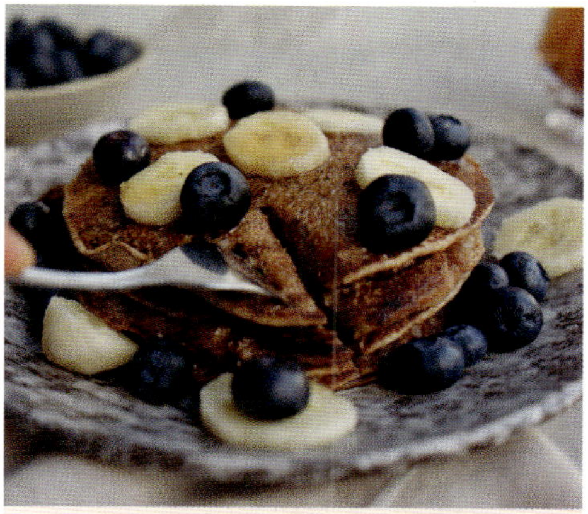

IN THE KITCHEN

B6 BREAKFAST

Start your day with homemade wheat bran pancakes served with banana and blueberries, accompanied with a glass of milk.

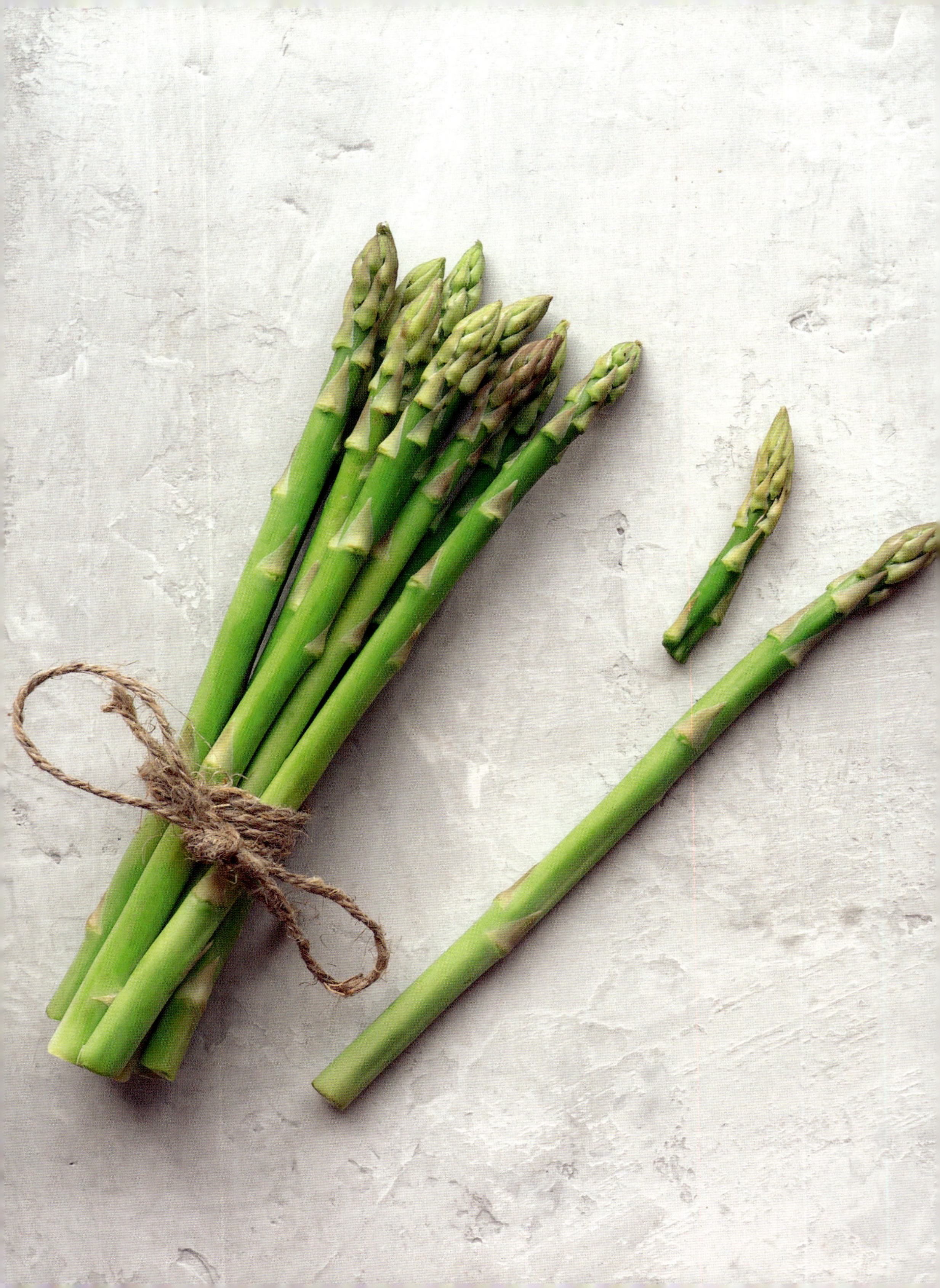

[VITAMIN B9]

- FOLATE -

THE **FOLIAGE** VITAMIN

RECOMMENDED DIETARY ALLOWANCE (RDA)

Men and women	400 mcg DFE
Pregnancy	600 mcg DFE
Lactation	500 mcg DFE

DFE: dietary folate equivalents

If you have ever taken prenatal vitamins, then you are likely aware of the importance of folate for healthy pregnancies.

FOLATE AND FOLIC ACID

Folate, sometimes called vitamin B9, is a water-soluble nutrient that is extremely important for proper nervous system and spinal cord development in utero.

But folate also has many important functions in the human body throughout the lifecycle, including assisting with amino acid metabolism. Along with vitamins B6 and B12, folate plays a role in the regulation of homocysteine levels in the blood.

As its name suggests, the best source of folate in the diet is "foliage," or green leafy vegetables. Folate also exists in its synthetic form, folic acid, in supplements and fortified foods. Therefore, the RDAs for folate are given as DFEs to account for both folate and folic acid. Due to differences in chemical structure, folic acid is more bioavailable than folate.

COMMON FOOD SOURCES

Folate can be found in leafy greens, legumes, and vegetables; folic acid is added to fortified cereals and enriched pasta. Incorporate enriched grains, spinach, lentils, and other beans in your weekly diet to meet your needs.

Lentils (1/2 cup, cooked)	179 mcg
Asparagus (8 spears, boiled)	178 mcg
White rice (1 cup, enriched, cooked)	153 mcg
Black beans (1 cup, canned)	146 mcg
Spinach (1/2 cup, boiled)	131 mcg
Spaghetti (1/2 cup, cooked)	74 mcg
Avocado (1/2 cup, sliced)	59 mcg
Mustard greens (1/2 cup, boiled)	52 mcg
Kidney beans (1/2 cup, canned)	46 mcg
Tomato juice (3/4 cup)	36 mcg

USING SUPPLEMENTS

Folic acid is one of the most common forms of folate available in supplements—on its own or as part of multivitamins, B-complex vitamins, and prenatal vitamins. Most adults consume enough folate from their diets. The UL for folic acid is 1,000 mcg per day.

ROLE IN THE BODY

Folate forms part of the important coenzymes that regulate cell division. This is why the demand for folate is so high during pregnancy, a time when there is rapid cell replication in fetal and maternal tissue.

Due to the role of folate in regulating blood levels of homocysteine, folate deficiency may be involved in the development of heart disease. As discussed on page 48, homocysteine is a protein that can increase the risk of heart disease when present in elevated levels in the blood. Vitamins B6 and B12 also play a role in regulating homocysteine, but studies suggest that increasing folate intake has the greatest effect on lowering homocysteine levels when there is no deficiency of these other vitamins. However, it's still unclear as to whether decreasing homocysteine concentrations in the blood actually reduces the risk of heart disease.

Folate is also vital to DNA and RNA methylation, or the process in which methyl groups are added to change the activity and gene expression of DNA and RNA. Issues with DNA methylation may lead to underlying damages that have been associated with cancer development. While more research is needed, some observational studies suggest that folate deficiency may be linked to some cancers.

NOTES ON DEFICIENCY

Similar to other B vitamins, folate deficiency rarely occurs on its own and typically happens at the same time as other deficiencies. Poor dietary intake, heavy alcohol consumption, and nutrient malabsorption can lead to deficiencies of folate and other nutrients. Signs of deficiency may include tongue ulcers, changes in skin, hair, and nail pigmentation, and high blood homocysteine levels.

Caution in pregnancy

Inadequate folate status during pregnancy increases the risk of neural tube defects in infants. Due to the increased demand for folate during pregnancy, pregnant women and all women of childbearing age need to be wary of consuming enough folate or folic acid from foods and supplements.

Megaloblastic anemia

Folate deficiency leads to megaloblastic anemia, marked by large and abnormal red blood cells and symptoms such as fatigue, heart palpitations, irritability, and shortness of breath. Folic acid supplementation typically resolves this condition. However, megaloblastic anemia can also result from vitamin B12 deficiency. It's important to properly identify the cause of megaloblastic anemia to avoid supplementing with the incorrect vitamin (see also, page 56).

DID YOU KNOW?

When scientists isolated it from spinach in 1941, folate was named after the word folium, *the Latin word for leaf.*

VIT TIPS

Increase your folate intake by adding more veggies to your meals. Start the day with a spinach and avocado smoothie, make a salad with lentils for lunch, and serve asparagus as a side with dinner.

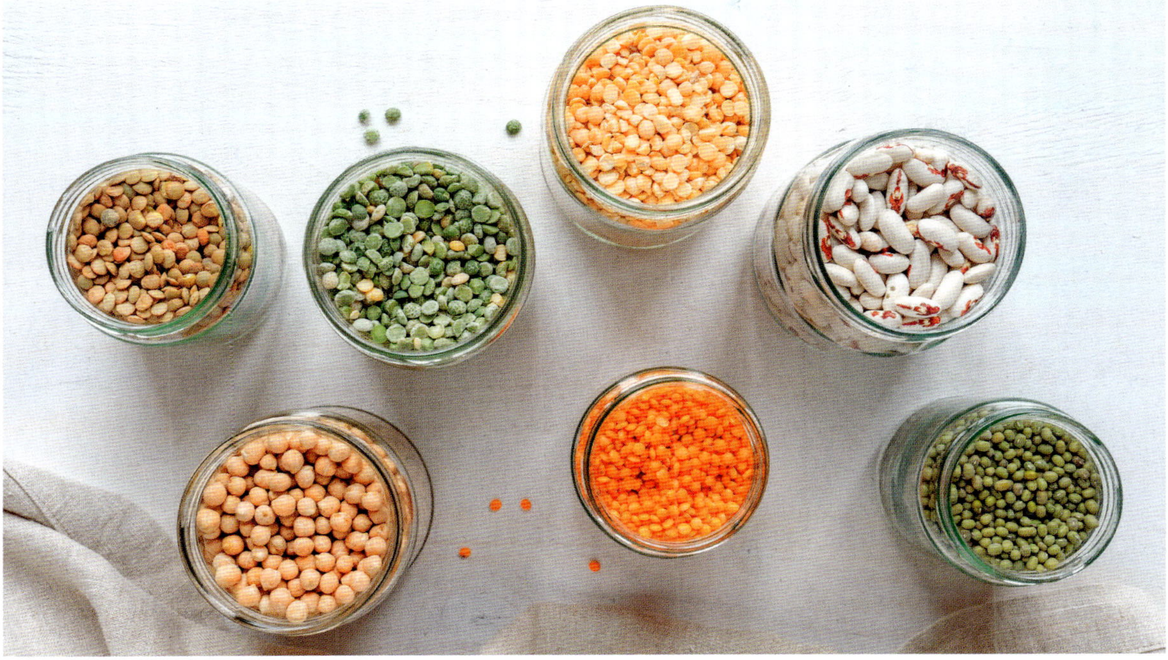

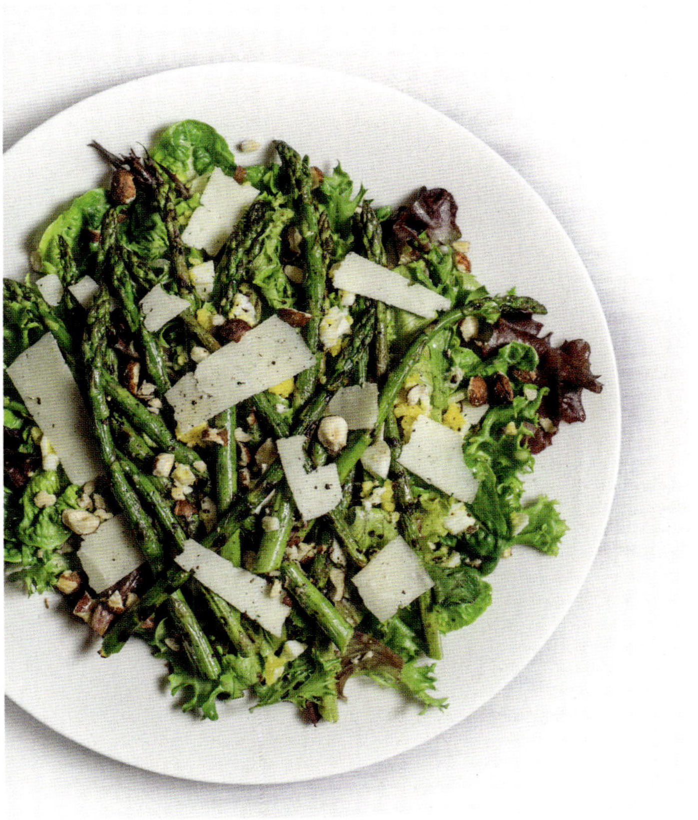

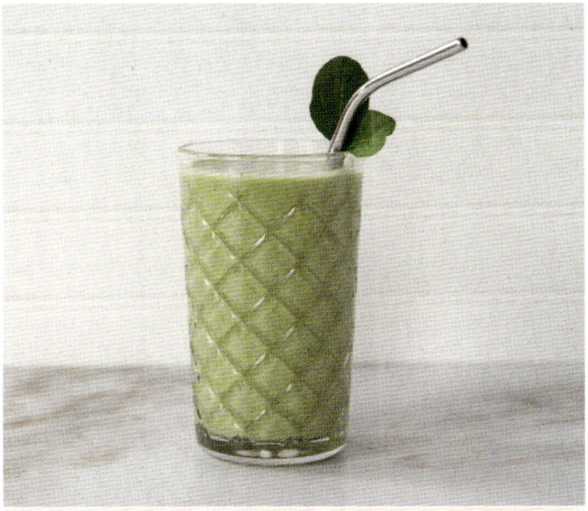

IN THE KITCHEN

FRUITY GREEN SMOOTHIE

To make a folate-rich smoothie, blend 2 cups raw spinach with ½ avocado, 1 cup frozen mango, a squeeze of lime juice, and water as needed.

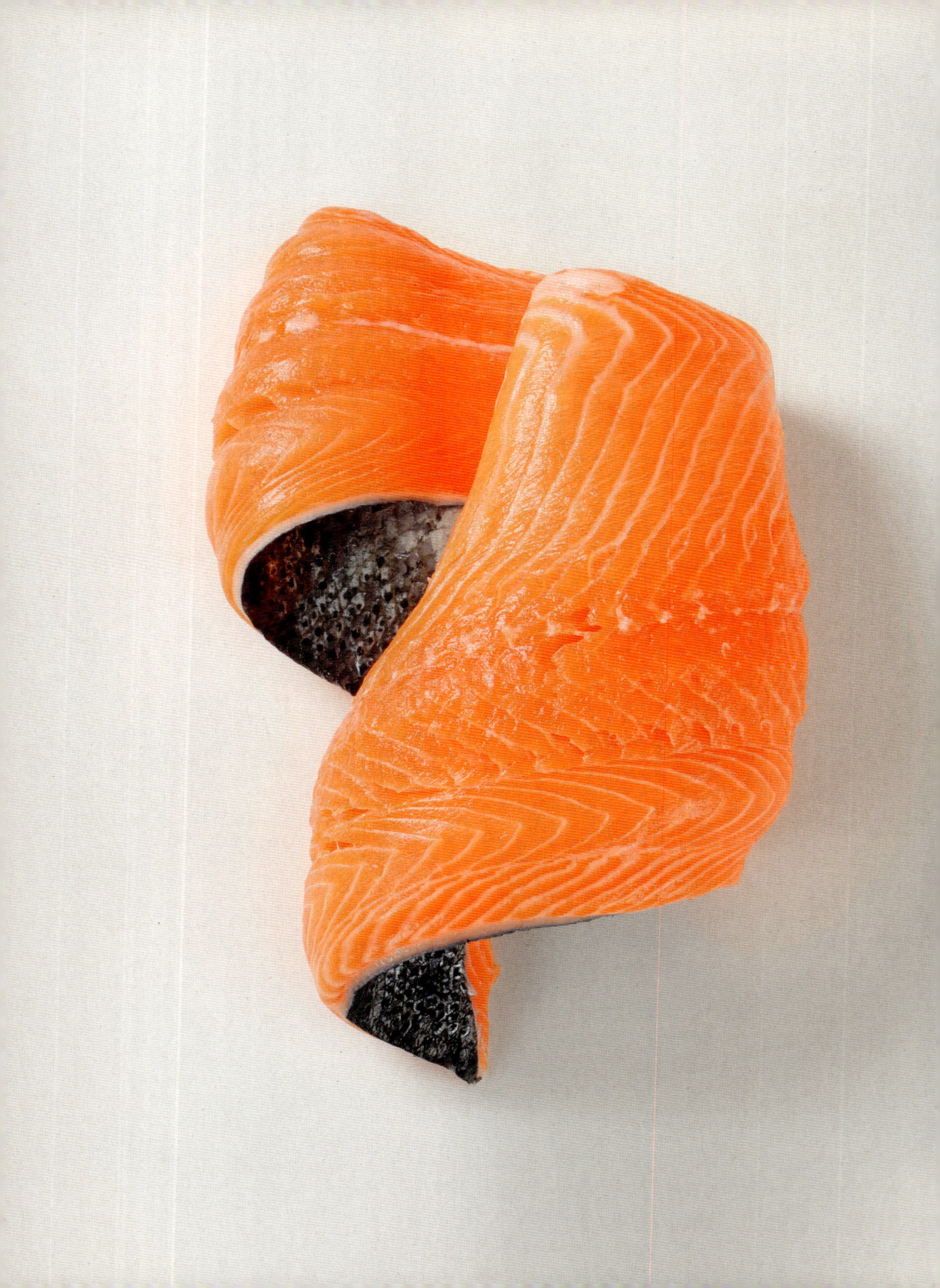

[VITAMIN B12]

- COBALAMIN -

THE NERVOUS SYSTEM **PROTECTOR**

RECOMMENDED DIETARY ALLOWANCE (RDA)

Men and women	2.4 mcg*
Pregnancy	2.6 mcg
Lactation	2.8 mcg

*While the RDA for adults is 2.4 mcg, some experts suggest that individuals 51 years of age and older take B12 supplements in higher doses, since B12 absorption may decrease with age.

The discovery of water-soluble vitamin B12 began in 1849, when Dr. Thomas Addison (the same physician credited with discovering Addison's disease) started to see a terrible kind of anemia in patients.

HISTORIC FINDINGS

In 1872, Dr. Antoine Biemer coined the disease "pernicious anemia" since it often led to death. Eventually, anemia due to B12 deficiency was easy to treat and no longer fatal, thanks in part to Nobel-winning experiments that involved feeding patients large amounts of liver.

The interesting history of vitamin B12 paints the picture of what we know about this nutrient today. The term vitamin B12 refers to several compounds that have similar activity in the body and play a role in nerve function and the creation of red blood cells. Since they contain the mineral cobalt, vitamin B12 is also called cobalamin. As the historical experiments with liver suggest, vitamin B12 naturally occurs in animal, but not plant, foods. Vitamin B12 deficiency is often a concern for those who follow a vegan or vegetarian diet, as well as older adults and individuals who have limited absorption of the nutrient.

COMMON FOOD SOURCES

Vitamin B12 is added to several fortified foods in bioavailable forms, and is bound to protein in foods. Just three ounces of smoked salmon provides more than a day's worth of B12.

Clams (3 oz, cooked)	84 mcg
Beef liver (3 oz, cooked)	71 mcg
Smoked salmon (3 oz)	2.8 mcg
Nutritional yeast fortified with 100% of the RDA (1 serving)	2.4 mcg
Skim milk (1 cup)	0.9 mcg
Turkey (3 oz, roasted)	0.8 mcg
Breakfast cereal fortified with 25% of the RDA (1 serving)	0.6 mcg
Egg (1 large, poached)	0.4 mcg

USING SUPPLEMENTS

Most adults consume enough B12 in their diets. Supplements often contain cyanocobalamin, which is converted into active forms of B12 in the body. For those avoiding animal products, vegan-friendly supplements exist, and there are injections and patches for those with absorption issues. It is not considered toxic in high doses and there is no UL.

ROLE IN THE BODY

Vitamin B12 is largely important to nerve function, homocysteine metabolism, DNA synthesis, and the creation of red blood cells. Specifically, it helps preserve the protective coating around nervous system and brain cells called myelin sheath. This function has led to speculation about the protective role of vitamin B12 in Alzheimer's disease. Some research suggests that vitamin B12 deficiency is associated with this disease, but more studies are needed.

Cobalamin is a cofactor for an enzyme involved in the creation of hemoglobin, the protein in red blood cells that carries oxygen throughout the body. It's also required for the proper functioning of an enzyme that plays a role in DNA and RNA methylation. Together with folate and vitamin B6, it regulates blood homocysteine levels and prevents accumulation of this protein, which has been linked to heart disease.

NOTES ON DEFICIENCY

One of the most common causes of vitamin B12 deficiency is impaired absorption, as opposed to inadequate dietary intake. Vitamin B12 absorption requires intrinsic factor, a protein secreted by the stomach. Pernicious anemia can result from an autoimmune disease or the surgical removal of portions of the stomach, which inhibits the production of intrinsic factor, leading to vitamin B12 deficiency and megaloblastic anemia.

Who's at risk?

Individuals with digestive disorders, including celiac and Crohn's disease, have a higher risk of developing vitamin B12 deficiency. Older adults are also at increased risk, since they may be more likely to have gastritis and stomach inflammation that inhibits vitamin B12 absorption.

What are the symptoms?

Symptoms of B12 deficiency include megaloblastic anemia, marked by fatigue and irritability, neurological changes, such as numbness and tingling in the hands and feet, confusion, depression, and poor memory. Deficiency is often treated with high doses of oral supplements and/or intramuscular B12 injections that are more effective for people with absorption issues.

DID YOU KNOW?

The body's vitamin B12 stores can last up to five years, so deficiency may take a long time to develop, even in individuals with inadequate intake.

VIT TIPS

Vegans looking to boost their B12 intake can try air-popped popcorn sprinkled with salt and fortified nutritional yeast, a yellow, deactivated yeast that has a cheesy flavor.

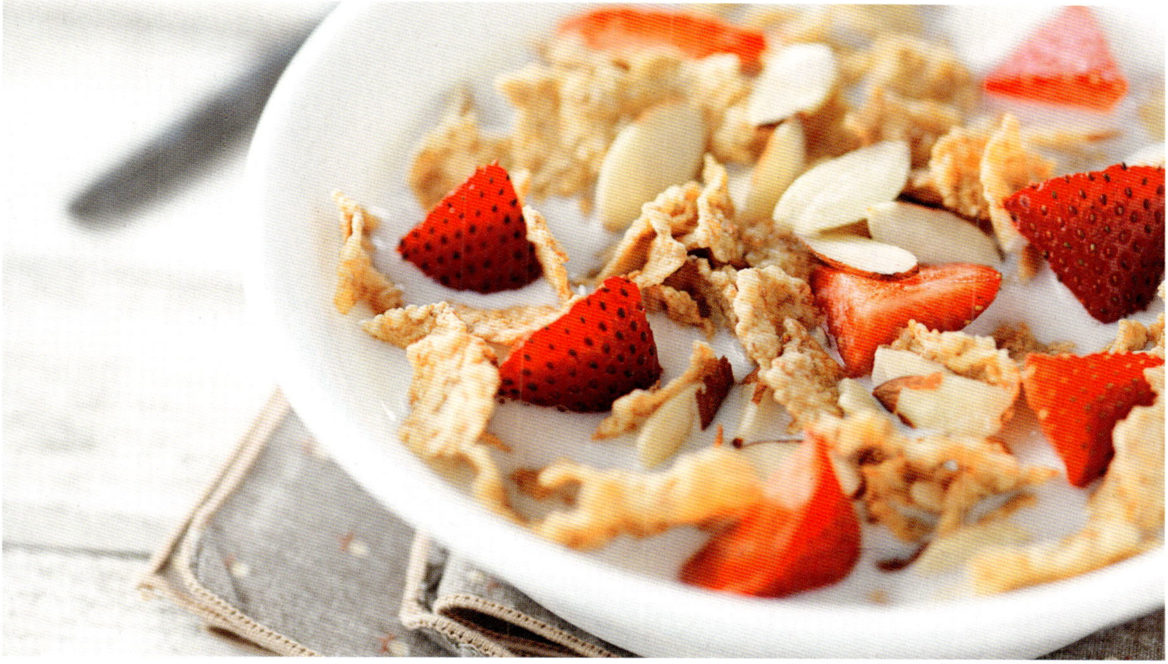

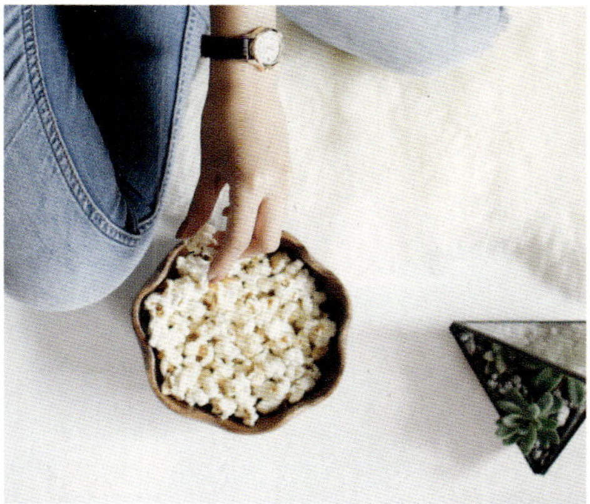

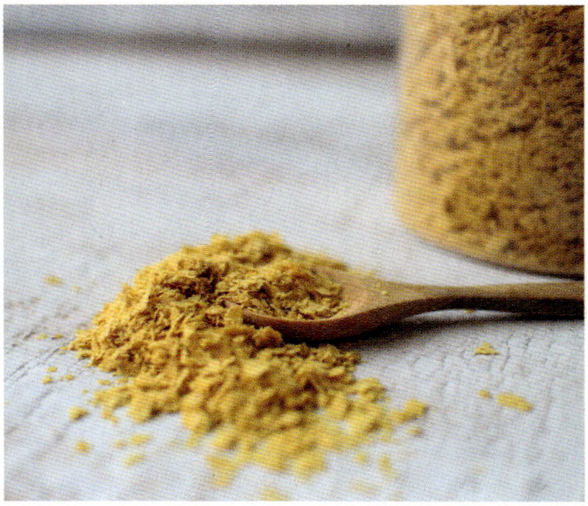

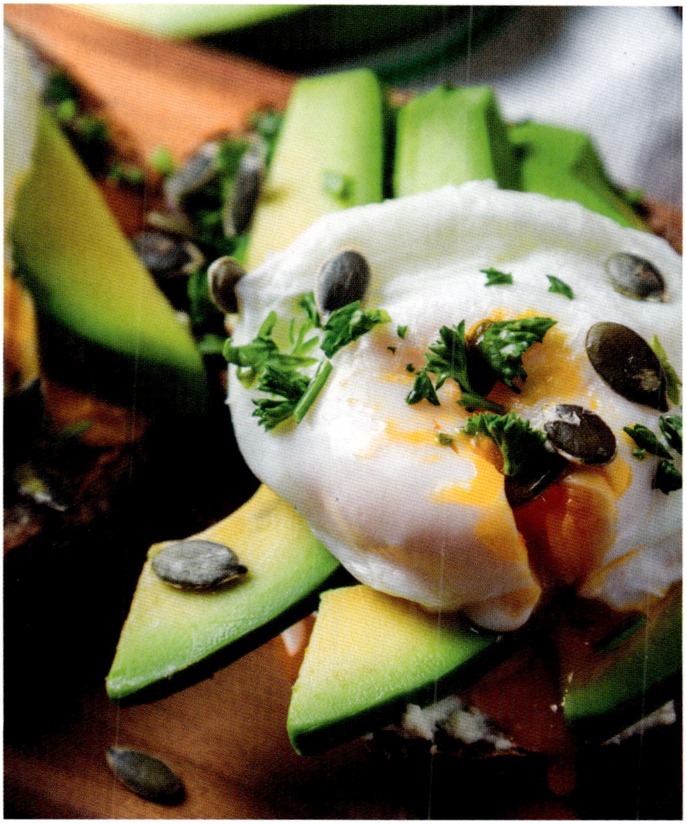

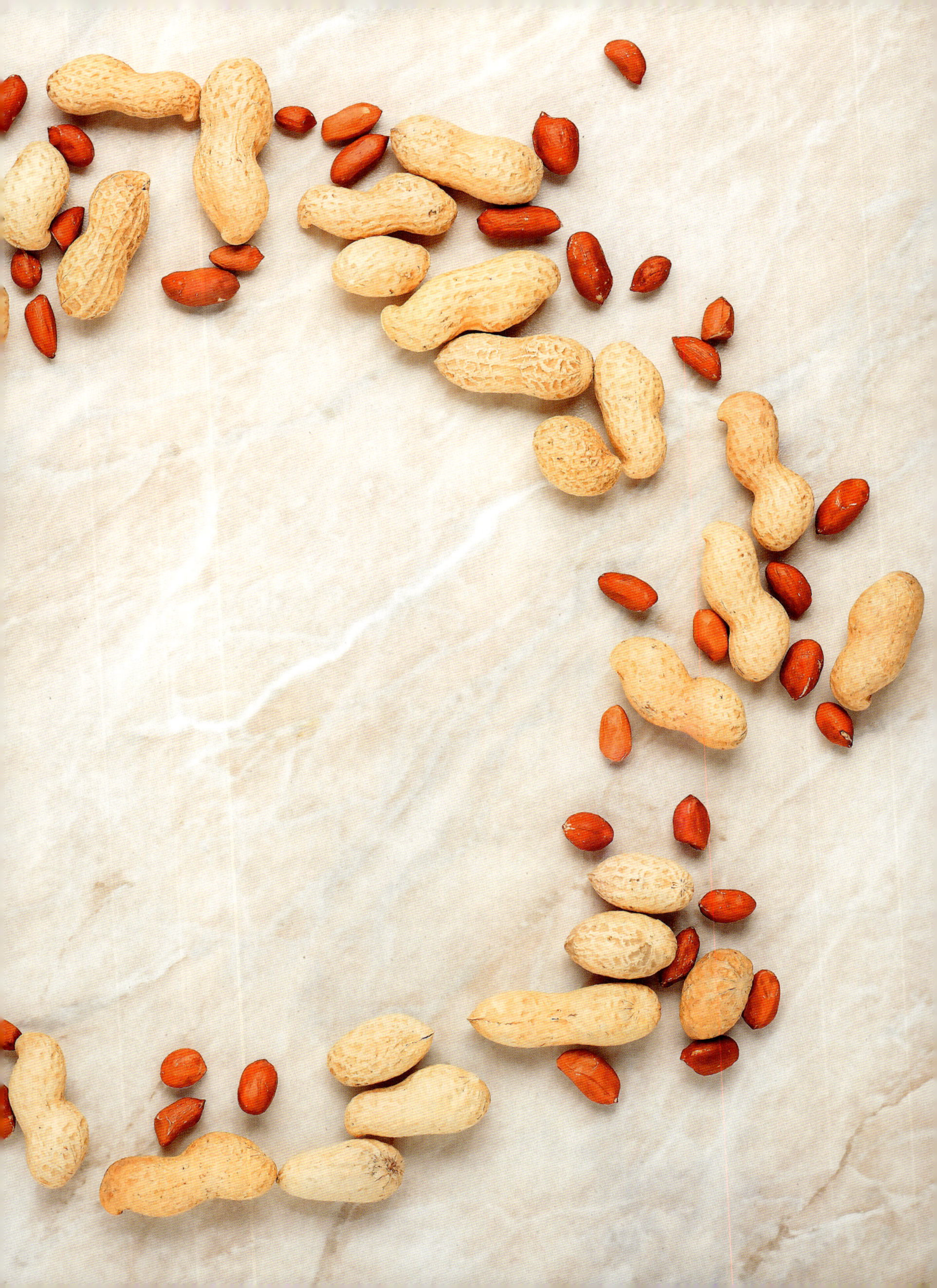

[BIOTIN]

ADEQUATE INTAKE (AI)

Men and women	30 mcg
Pregnancy	30 mcg
Lactation	35 mcg

THE **BEAUTY** VITAMIN

Beauty supplements and products often portray biotin as the key to glossy hair, healthy nails, and glowing skin. While these claimed benefits may be familiar to you, you may not know the history behind them.

ALL ABOUT BIOTIN

It was first discovered that humans needed biotin, a water-soluble B vitamin, after experiments that involved feeding rats egg-white protein led to hair loss and severe skin inflammation. Raw egg whites have a protein that binds to biotin, therefore preventing absorption and highlighting the effects of biotin deficiency. Biotin also plays a key role in gene expression and the production of energy from fats, carbohydrates, and proteins.

COMMON FOOD SOURCES

Biotin is found in many different foods. While it is true that eating lots of raw egg whites can inhibit biotin absorption, cooked eggs are not a problem and are actually one of the best sources of this nutrient. A three-egg omelet provides enough biotin for the whole day. On days when you don't eat eggs, meet your needs with plant-based sources of biotin.

Egg (1 large, cooked)	10 mcg
Avocado (1 fruit, cubed)	2–6 mcg
Peanuts (1 oz, roasted)	5 mcg
Pork chop (3 oz, cooked)	3.8 mcg
Hamburger patty (3 oz, cooked)	3.8 mcg
Sweet potato (1/2 cup, cooked)	2.4 mcg
Raspberries (1 cup, raw)	0.2–2 mcg
Almonds (1/4 cup, roasted)	1.5 mcg
Spinach (1/2 cup, boiled)	0.4 mcg

USING SUPPLEMENTS

Healthy adults who eat a varied diet do not need biotin supplements. In fact, there is minimal research that backs the claims that biotin supplements promote hair, skin, and nail health.

ROLE IN THE BODY

The main function of biotin is a cofactor for five carboxylases, enzymes that regulate the metabolism of food components: fatty acids, glucose, and amino acids. In other words, biotin is vital for converting food into usable energy.

Biotin may also promote health and help prevent disease, but the role of this nutrient in overall health is less clear. The symptoms of biotin deficiency suggest that biotin is necessary for healthy skin, hair, and nails, but only a few, non-controlled studies have found that biotin supplements increase nail thickness in those with brittle or thin fingernails. There are almost no published studies on the impact of biotin on skin and hair in healthy individuals.

Another area of interest is the use of biotin supplements in improving motor function impairments in patients with multiple sclerosis (MS). The promising results of preliminary studies have led to ongoing trials that are evaluating the potential role of biotin in MS treatment.

DID YOU KNOW?

There have been no reported cases of toxicity with biotin supplements up to 200 mg orally and 50 mg intravenously.

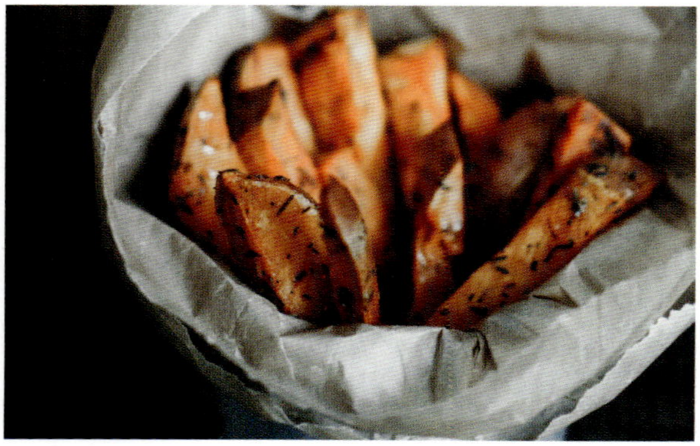

NOTES ON DEFICIENCY

It is highly unlikely that an individual eating a varied diet would develop biotin deficiency. However, individuals with alcoholism may have impaired biotin absorption and status. Pregnant and breastfeeding women may also be at risk of inadequate intake, especially since biotin levels decrease during lactation.

VIT TIPS

Breastfeeding moms need an extra 5 mcg of biotin per day, which is just about the amount in a cup of cooked sweet potato.

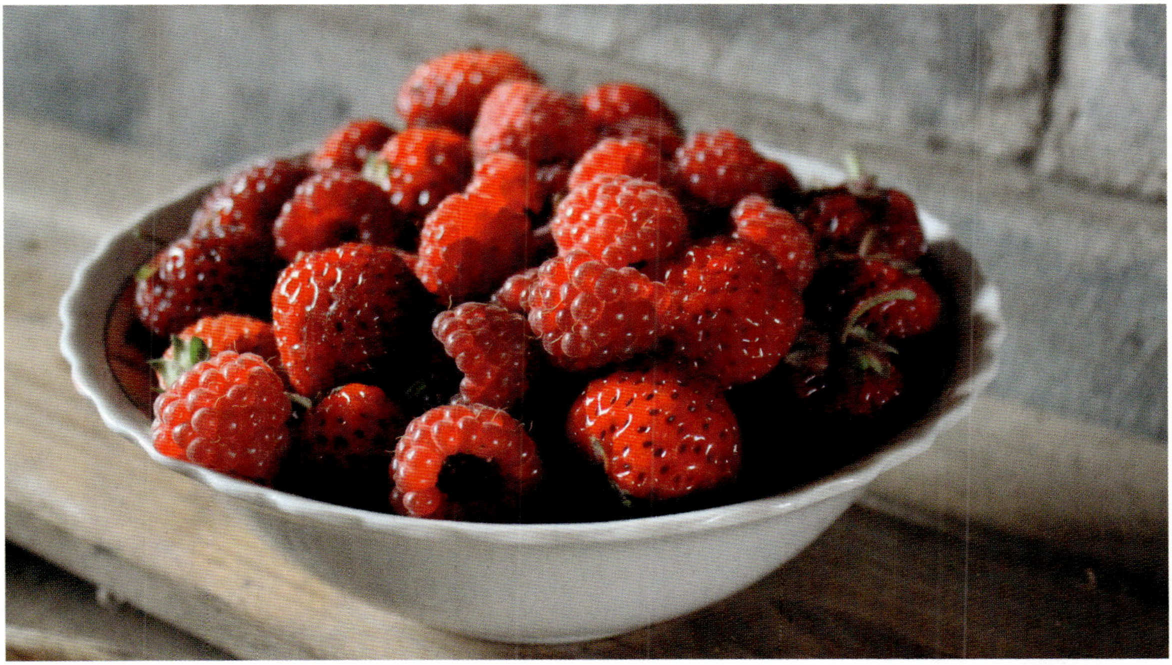

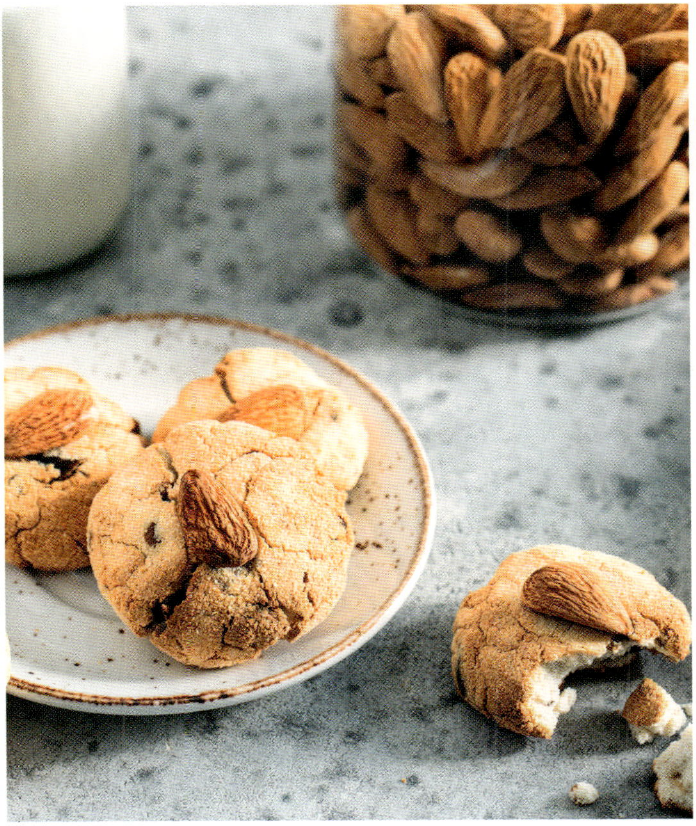

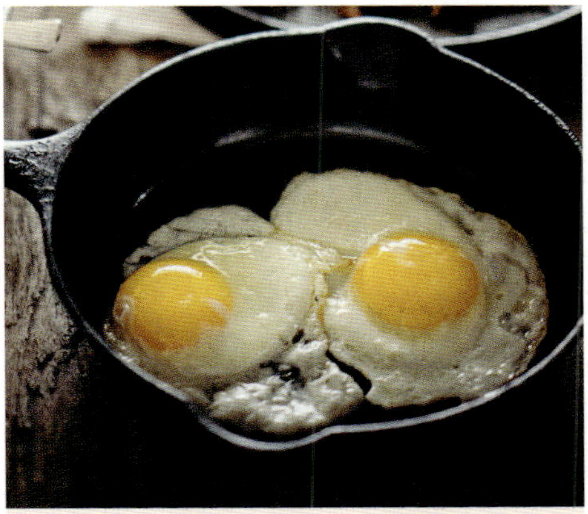

IN THE KITCHEN

BIOTIN BOOSTER

Dish up a bowl of roasted sweet potatoes, topped with avocado and spinach and finished with a couple fried eggs.

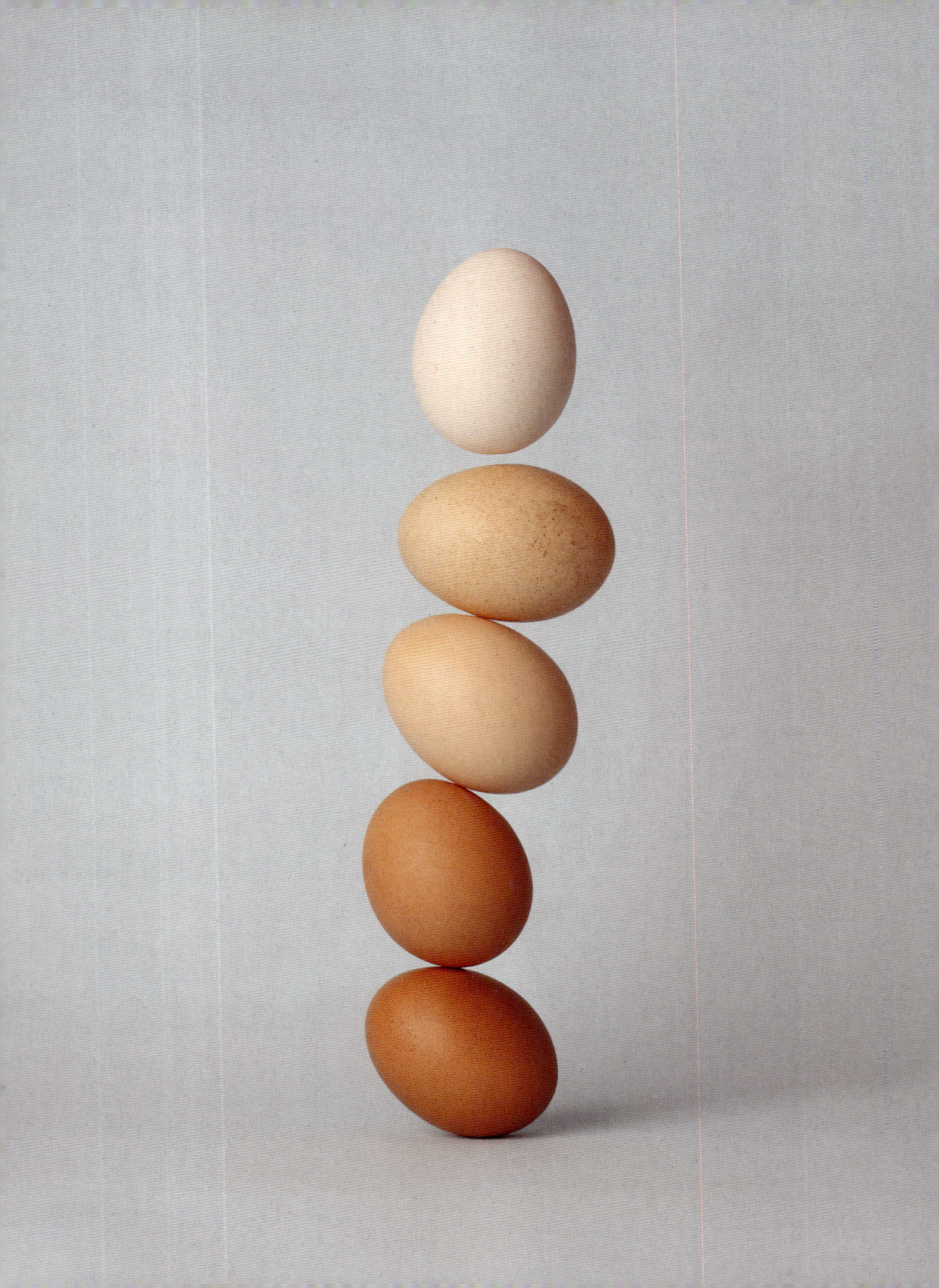

[CHOLINE]

ADEQUATE INTAKE (AI)

Men	550 mg
Women	425 mg
Pregnancy	450 mg
Lactation	550 mg

THE LIVER **PROTECTOR**

Choline is an essential vitamin-like nutrient that you must get from your diet, but it is not technically a vitamin.

ALL ABOUT CHOLINE

Since some of the functions of choline are similar to those of other B vitamins, such as lipid metabolism and methylation reactions, it's frequently grouped with them in nutrition discussions.

It was originally thought that the body could synthesize enough choline to support its many functions, but scientists eventually discovered that this is not the case. The possible health benefits of choline continue to be explored, especially in relation to brain development, dementia, and heart and liver health. Choline is often discussed in regards to pregnancy, when the need for this nutrient likely increases.

COMMON FOOD SOURCES

Even though the body can make choline, it can't produce enough to support health. It's vital to get adequate choline from food sources, especially during pregnancy. Incorporating the foods on this list into your weekly diet will help you meet your needs.

Egg (1 large, hard-boiled)	147 mg
Soybeans (1/2 cup, roasted)	107 mg
Chicken breast (3 oz, roasted)	72 mg
Lean ground beef (3 oz, broiled)	72 mg
Cod (3 oz, cooked)	71 mg
Kidney beans (1/2 cup, canned)	45 mg
1% milk (1 cup)	43 mg
Brussels sprouts (1/2 cup, boiled)	32 mg
Shiitake mushrooms (1/2 cup, cooked)	27 mg
Cabbage (1/2 cup, boiled)	15 mg
Tangerine (1/2 cup of sections)	10 mg

USING SUPPLEMENTS

Research suggests that most people don't consume enough choline from their diets, but deficiency is still rare. Therefore, choline supplementation is not recommended unless there is a reason.

ROLE IN THE BODY

Choline is necessary for the creation of phospholipids, which provide structure to all cell membranes and takes part in the synthesis of myelin sheath that protects nerve cells. As its name suggests, the neurotransmitter acetylcholine is also made from choline. Acetylcholine plays a crucial role in muscle control and memory.

Deficiency of choline has been linked to nonalcoholic fatty liver disease (NAFLD) and liver damage, since choline is necessary for creating the carriers that transport fat and cholesterol out of the liver. Several studies suggest that adequate choline consumption may be an important aspect of preventing NAFLD.

Other functions of choline include acting as a source of methyl groups in the methylation of homocysteine, a process discussed on pages 52 and 56. It also plays a role in the reabsorption of water in the kidneys.

NOTES ON DEFICIENCY

Overt choline deficiency is rare, but can lead to muscle and liver damage, as well as NAFLD. On the other hand, inadequate choline intake is very common. It's estimated that 90–95% of pregnant women do not get enough choline, and most prenatal supplements do not include this nutrient. Some research suggests that low choline levels during pregnancy can increase the risk of neural tube defects in infants, but other studies offer conflicting results. Finally, patients receiving total parenteral nutrition (TPN) are at increased risk of choline deficiency.

DID YOU KNOW?

Choline was discovered in 1862 but not recognized as an essential nutrient until 1998, more than 135 years later.

VIT TIPS

Getting too much choline from supplements or food can lead to fishy body odor and low blood pressure. The UL for choline is set at 3,500 mg per day for adults.

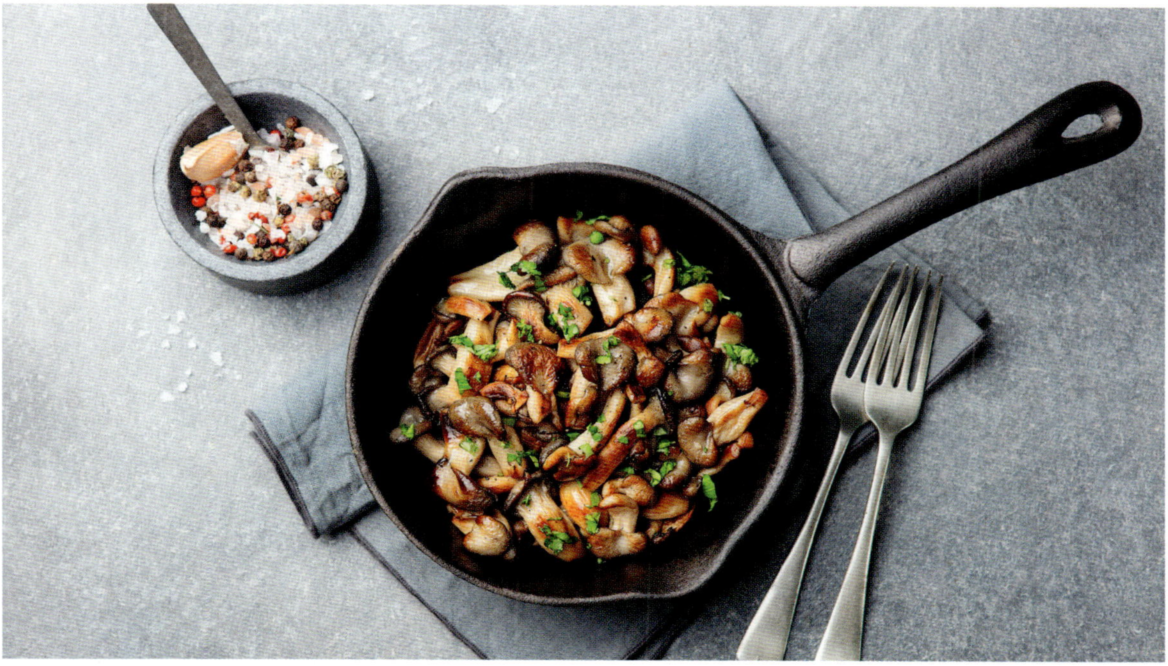

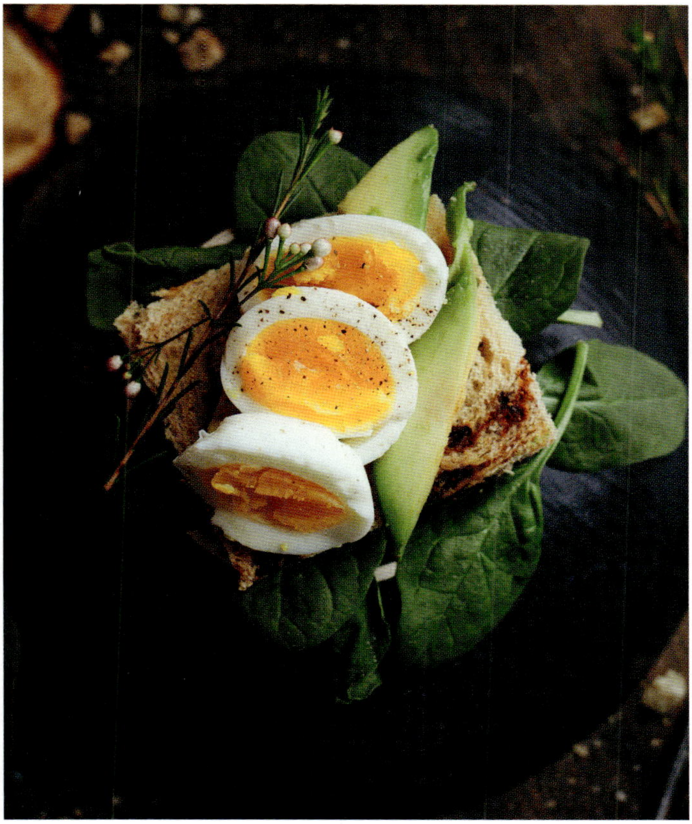

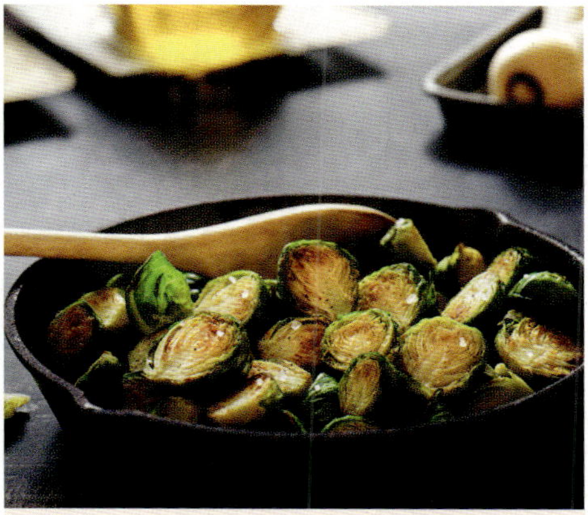

IN THE KITCHEN

SPROUTS SIDE

Meet your choline needs by serving a generous spoonful of Brussels sprouts with peanut-crusted chicken and sautéed mushrooms on the side.

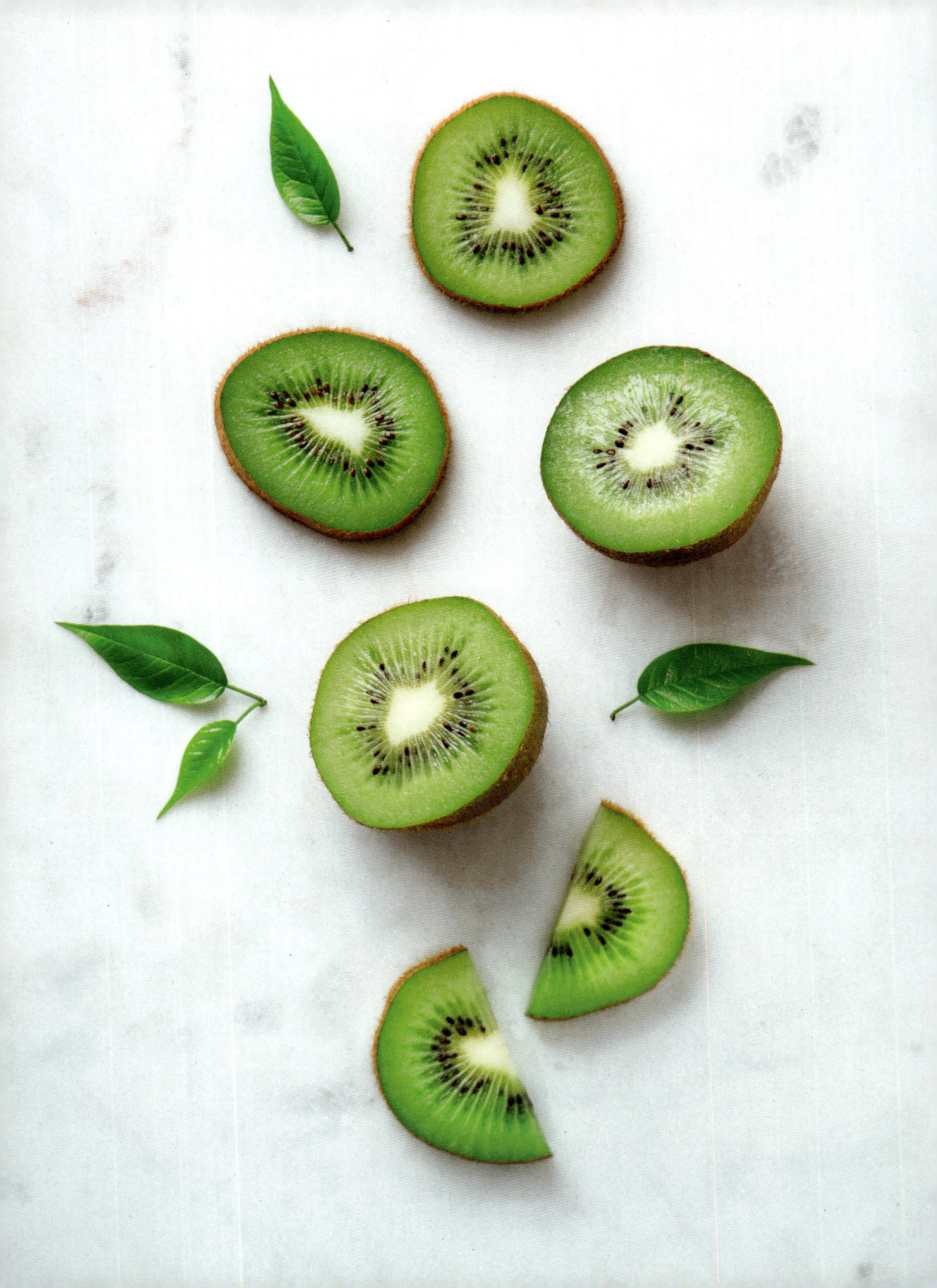

[VITAMIN C]

- ASCORBIC ACID -

THE **POWERFUL** ANTIOXIDANT

RECOMMENDED DIETARY ALLOWANCE (RDA)

Men	90 mg
Women	75 mg
Pregnancy (14–18 years)	80 mg
Pregnancy (19+ years)	85 mg
Lactation (14–18 years)	115 mg
Lactation (19+ years)	120 mg
Smokers	35 mg more than nonsmokers

Vitamin C has become almost synonymous with immune function, but do you know about its many other functions?

ALL ABOUT ASCORBIC ACID

This water-soluble nutrient, also known as L-ascorbic acid, is a powerful antioxidant that may protect against certain chronic diseases. It's necessary for the creation of collagen, the most abundant fibrous protein in the body, and it even helps with the absorption of nonheme iron (see page 113).

Vitamin C exists in many foods, but it can be reduced during prolonged storage and cooking. Fresh, raw fruits and vegetables will typically provide more vitamin C than cooked ones.

USING SUPPLEMENTS

Limited evidence suggests that supplements may decrease the duration of the common cold but they do not protect you from getting sick in the first place. Although not considered toxic, high supplemental intake may lead to diarrhea. The UL is 2,000 mg per day.

COMMON FOOD SOURCES

While you may think of oranges as the best source of vitamin C, numerous fruits and vegetables contain this nutrient. In fact, one medium kiwi has almost the same amount of vitamin C as a medium orange. Each of these fruits provides close to the RDA for vitamin C, but if you don't like those options, 1/2 cup of red bell pepper has more than enough vitamin C for the whole day.

Red bell pepper (1/2 cup, raw)	95 mg
Orange (1 medium)	70 mg
Kiwi (1 medium)	64 mg
Broccoli (1/2 cup, cooked)	51 mg
Strawberries (1/2 cup, sliced)	49 mg
Brussels sprouts (1/2 cup, cooked)	48 mg
Grapefruit (1/2 medium)	39 mg
Tomato juice (3/4 cup)	33 mg
Cantaloupe (1/2 cup)	29 mg
Cauliflower (1/2 cup, raw)	26 mg
Yukon gold potatoes (2/3 cup, mashed)	21 mg

ROLE IN THE BODY

The best-known function of vitamin C is its pivotal role in immune health. In addition to acting as an antioxidant and preventing free radical damage to immune cells, vitamin C enhances the production of white blood cells. While it's clear that vitamin C is necessary for the functioning of the immune system, it's a bit of a stretch to refer to it as an "immune booster."

Current research offers conflicting results as to whether vitamin C actually strengthens the immune system in the general population outside of the role in its basic functioning. However, vitamin C may boost immunity and reduce the risk of getting sick in individuals exposed to extreme exercise, stress, and cold environments, but more research is needed.

Vitamin C is also necessary for the creation of collagen, which makes up connective tissue and helps with wound healing. Finally, due to its role as an antioxidant, it's thought that vitamin C may help protect against heart disease, cancer, and other conditions that involve oxidative stress. Intravenous vitamin C is sometimes given to cancer patients to slow disease progression. While some research reports that these treatments lead to improved quality of life, the extent to which intravenous vitamin C fights cancer, or any disease, is unclear.

NOTES ON DEFICIENCY

True vitamin C deficiency leads to scurvy, characterized by poor wound healing, joint pain, and swollen, bleeding gums. Scurvy is very rare in the United States, but some populations are at risk of inadequate intake of vitamin C. These include smokers, who require more vitamin C because of increased oxidative stress, and those who eat a diet with very few fruits and vegetables.

DID YOU KNOW?

In the 1700s, British navy surgeon James Lind used citrus fruits to treat scurvy. It wasn't until 1932 that vitamin C was found to be responsible.

VIT TIPS

Vitamin C is water-soluble and destroyed by heat. Therefore, it's best to eat foods containing vitamin C raw or to prepare them by steaming or microwaving instead of using longer, higher heat cooking methods.

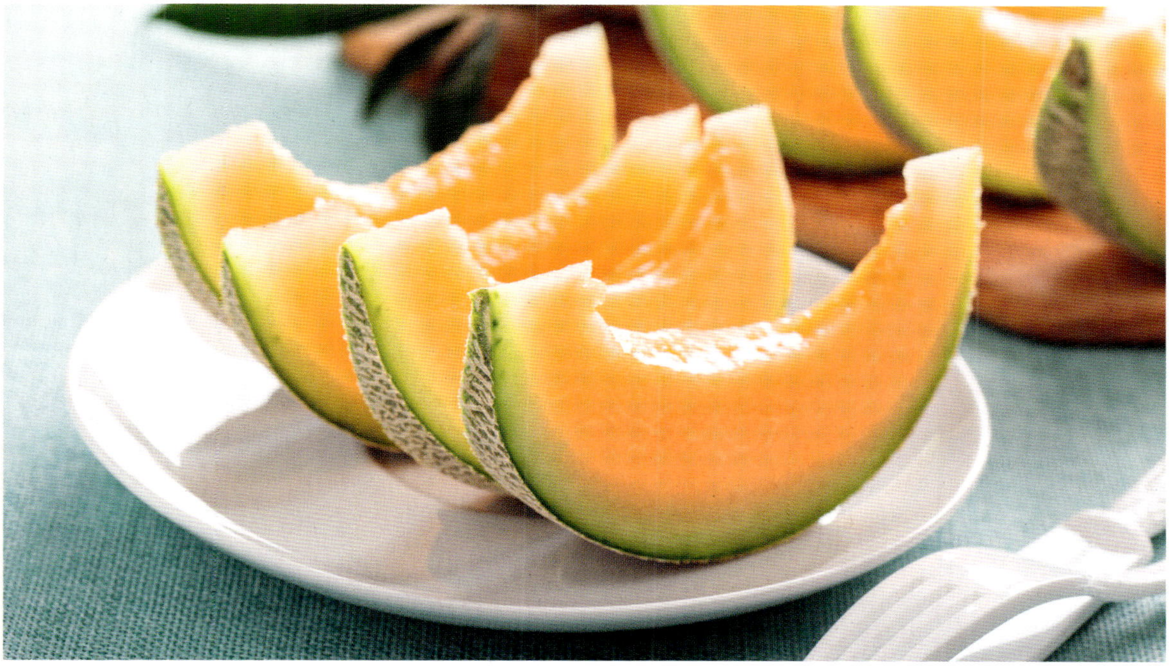

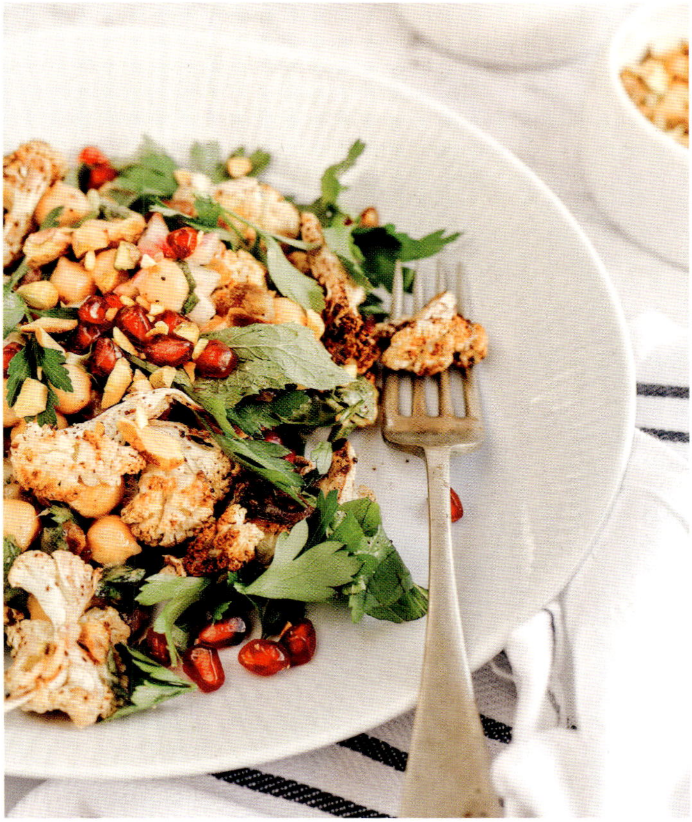

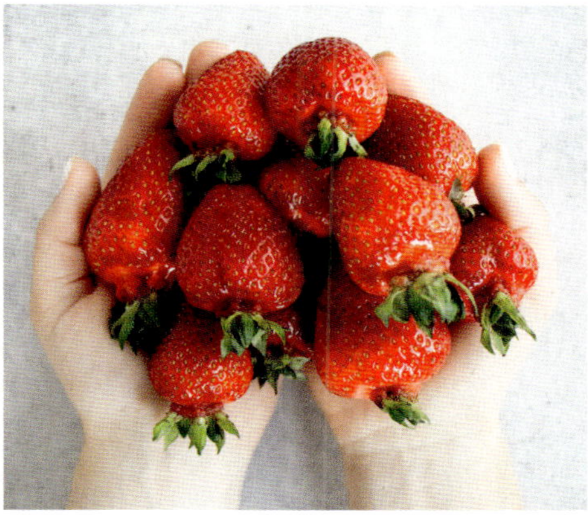

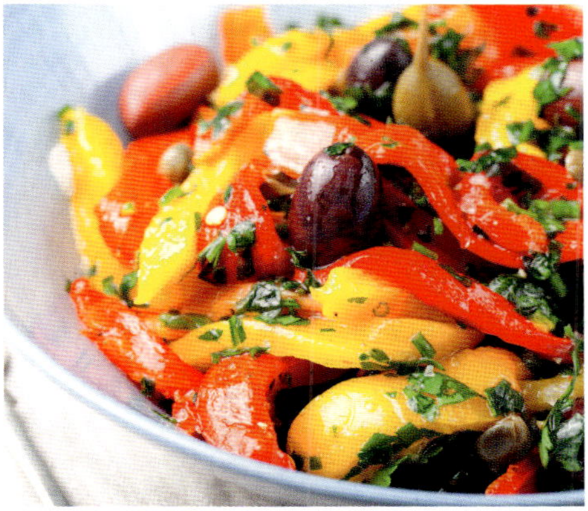

PART TWO: MINERALS

Each mineral plays a unique role in human health and is typically categorized as either a major or a trace mineral, depending on the amounts in which it is needed for health. Trace minerals are no less important than major minerals.

This chapter begins with calcium, the body's most abundant mineral, before diving into the electrolytes and other major minerals. The trace minerals also get their time to shine, with information about functions, benefits, deficiency, and the best dietary sources.

As you page through this section, check out the Mineral Tips and In the Kitchen ideas to see how you can meet your needs at home. The information can help you assess whether your intake of certain nutrients is adequate. If you still have questions about whether you need supplements or have signs of deficiency, be sure to discuss this with your physician.

DID YOU KNOW?

Minerals cannot be destroyed by heat or light and do not change during digestion. For this reason, cooking foods does not destroy minerals as it does to some vitamins. However, minerals can leach out of foods during boiling or when nutrient-rich juice seeps out of meats and other foods.

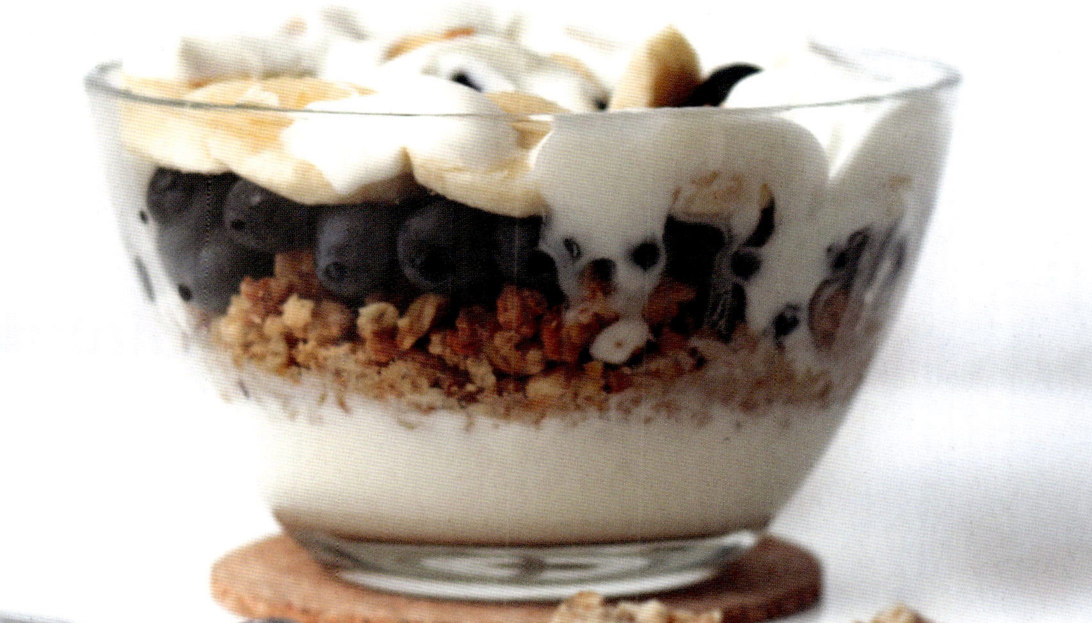

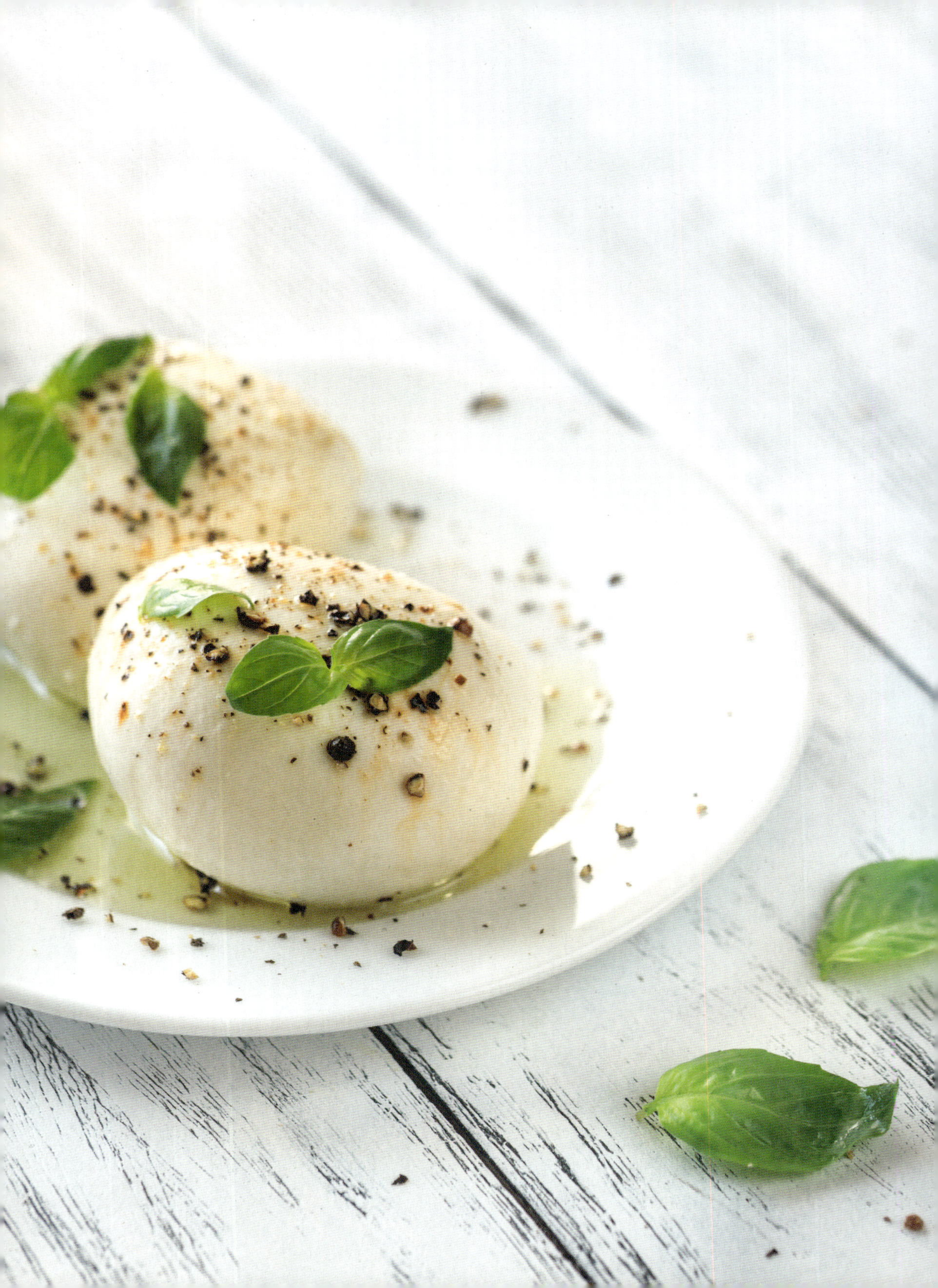

[CALCIUM]

THE BONE **BUILDER**

RECOMMENDED DIETARY ALLOWANCE (RDA)

Men and women (19–50 years)	1,000 mg
Men (51–70 years)	1,000 mg
Women (51–70 years)	1,200 mg
Men and women (71+ years)	1,200 mg
Pregnancy and lactation (14–18 years)	1,300 mg
Pregnancy and lactation (19–50 years)	1,000 mg

If you were around during the "got milk" campaign in the United States in the 1990s, then you are well aware that milk is often touted as a bone-building drink. Many commercials from this campaign connected drinking milk with strength and success, a claim that was personified by famous athletes, and not drinking milk with weak and fragile bones. These claims stemmed from the high amounts of calcium that milk provides, giving insight into the functions of this mineral.

USING SUPPLEMENTS

Supplements are only helpful for those who have a hard time meeting the RDA for calcium from foods. Since calcium supplements may cause gas, bloating, or constipation, it's often recommended to split doses up throughout the day and take them with meals. Getting too much calcium from supplements, but not foods, may increase the risk of kidney stones and heart disease. The UL for calcium is 2,500 mg for men and women ages 19–50, and 2,000 mg for adults over 51 years of age.

COMMON FOOD SOURCES

Dairy products are one of the best sources of calcium in the diet, but it's also found in many plants and fortified foods. However, calcium from certain plants, such as spinach and rhubarb, is not as well absorbed as calcium from kale, broccoli, and bok choy. Nonfat milk products have more calcium than those with higher fat contents. A cup of yogurt, a few ounces of cheese, and a cup of cooked kale together provide enough calcium to meet your daily needs.

Plain yogurt (1 cup, low-fat)	415 mg
Sardines (3.75 oz, canned in water, with bones, drained)	351 mg
Orange juice (1 cup, fortified)	349 mg
Cheddar cheese (1.5 oz)	307 mg
Soymilk (1 cup, fortified)	299 mg
Collard greens (1 cup, boiled)	268 mg
Firm tofu made with calcium sulfate (½ cup)	253 mg
Mozzarella (1-oz slice)	205 mg
Chia seeds (2 tbsp)	152 mg
Almonds (¼ cup, raw)	95 mg
Kale (1 cup, cooked)	94 mg
Orange (1 medium)	60 mg

ROLE IN THE BODY

Calcium's main function is providing structure to bones and teeth. In addition, it helps muscles contract, regulates nerve transmission, and maintains blood pressure and acid-base balance in the blood. Calcium is also necessary for activating vitamin K-dependent proteins, known as clotting factors, which promote blood clot formation.

Skeletal and muscle cells have calcium channels that open to let calcium into the cell to stimulate muscle contraction. These channels play a role in blood pressure regulation by controlling the contraction and dilation of blood vessels. In fact, calcium channel blockers are a common medication for high blood pressure. They work to lower blood pressure by blocking calcium from entering heart cells, therefore allowing blood vessels to open and relax.

Because calcium is vital to so many processes, it is tightly regulated in the blood with the aid of vitamin D. If blood levels of calcium are too low, vitamin D signals the breakdown of bones to release calcium. The importance of calcium has also made it a nutrient of interest in disease prevention. Studies have linked low calcium intake with a higher risk of osteoporosis, colorectal cancer, obesity, and high blood pressure. However, research on whether calcium supplements help with these issues is mixed.

NOTES ON DEFICIENCY

Calcium is abundant in the body and can be released from the skeleton when levels are low, so true calcium deficiency is rare. Vitamin D deficiency and low magnesium levels due to alcoholism can lead to low blood calcium.

Weak bones

Even without true deficiency, chronic inadequate intake can weaken the bones and has been linked to the development of osteoporosis. Getting enough calcium is particularly important for children and young adults to achieve peak bone mass and continues to be important later in life to prevent bone loss. Groups at risk of calcium inadequacy include postmenopausal women and vegetarians, vegans, or those with lactose intolerance who do not consume enough calcium-rich plant foods in place of dairy products.

DID YOU KNOW?

Ninety-nine percent of the body's calcium stores exist in the bones and teeth.

MINERAL TIPS

Plant-based "milks" made from nuts, oats, and soy often have less calcium than dairy products—even when fortified. If you don't consume dairy products, be sure to include a range of plant-based sources of calcium to meet your needs.

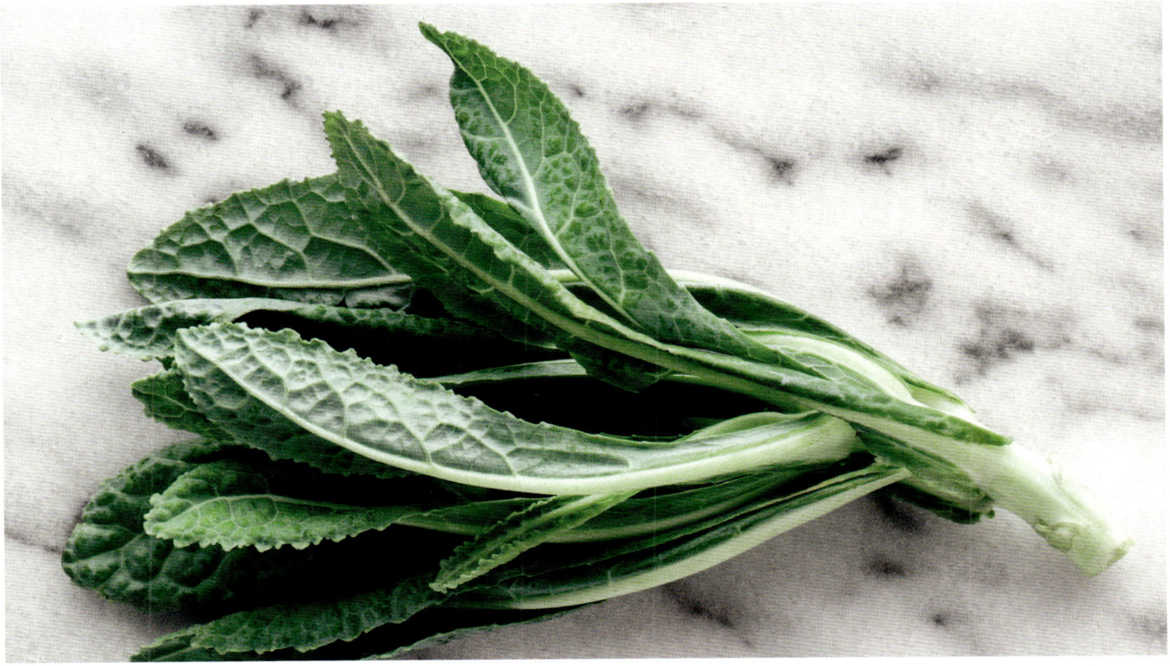

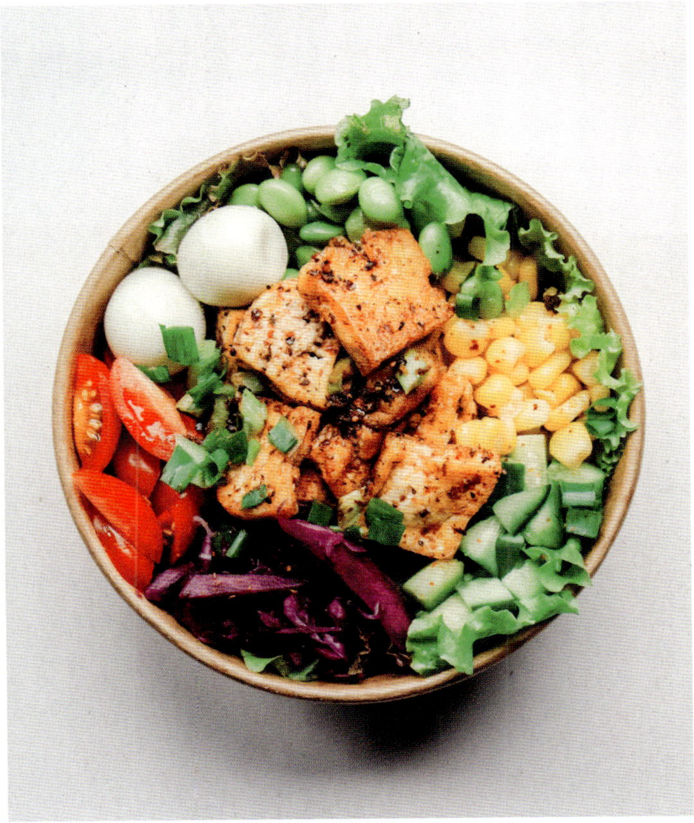

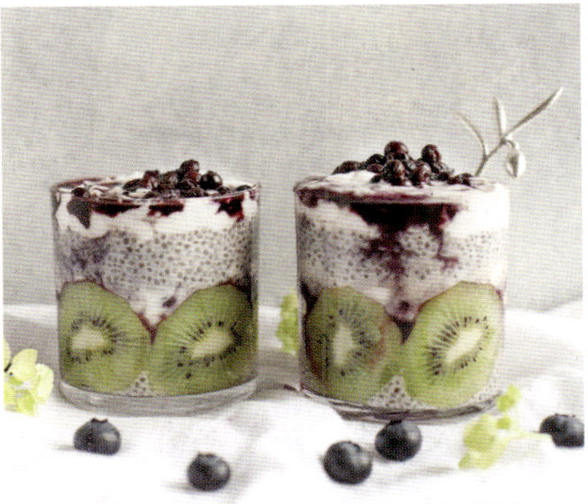

IN THE KITCHEN

CHIA SEED PUDDING

Try this delicious breakfast loaded with calcium. Mix 1 cup milk with 1 cup plain Greek yogurt, 1/4 cup chia seeds, 2 tbsp maple syrup, 1 tbsp vanilla extract, and a pinch of salt. Divide the pudding into small jars, seal, and pop in the fridge overnight to thicken. Serve with kiwi and blueberries.

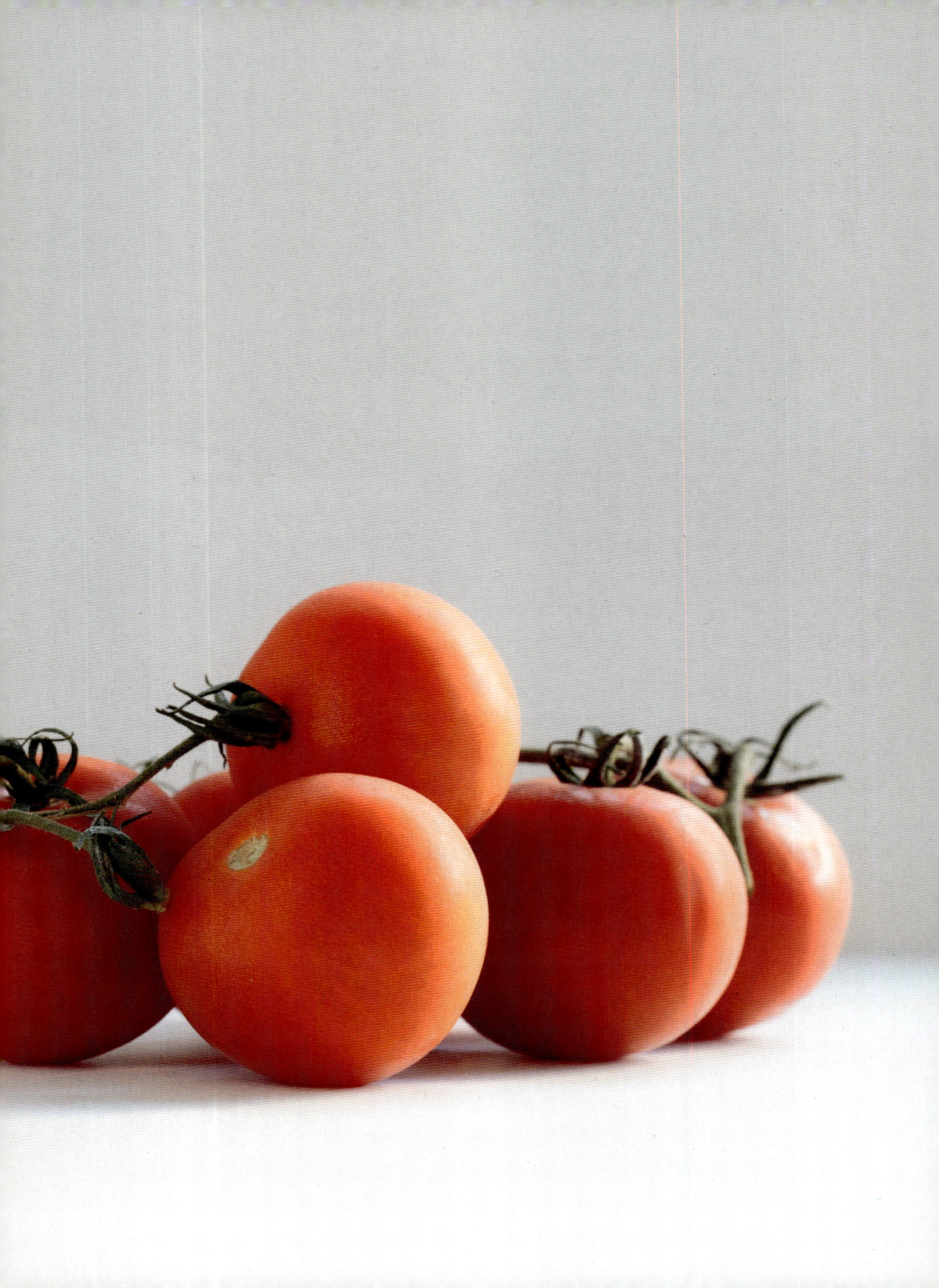

[CHLORIDE]

SODIUM'S **PARTNER**

ADEQUATE INTAKE (AI)

Men and women (18–50 years)	2,300 mg
Men and women (51–70 years)	2,000 mg
Men and women (71+ years)	1,800 mg
Pregnancy and lactation	2,300 mg

The functions of chloride are so connected to sodium, it's not typically discussed on its own. It still plays important roles in the body, however. Chloride is a major extracellular electrolyte, meaning that it is found in the fluid outside of cells. It helps to maintain the appropriate fluid volume and blood pressure.

COMMON FOOD SOURCES

The main source of chloride in the diet is salt, which is made up of sodium and chloride. Vegetables, including celery, tomatoes, and seaweed, have some naturally occurring chloride. Foods that are preserved with added salt, such as canned vegetables and processed meats, contain high amounts of chloride. Chloride is also one of the main ingredients in salt substitutes, along with the potassium that is used to replace salt (see page 91).

USING SUPPLEMENTS

It's unnecessary to take chloride supplements, since food sources provide plenty of this electrolyte.

ROLE IN THE BODY

Chloride is the most abundant negatively charged electrolyte in extracellular fluid. It works with sodium and potassium to maintain fluid volume and pressure.

Additionally, chloride plays an important role in maintaining the body's acid-base balance. Stomach cells need chloride to produce hydrochloric acid, a main component of digestive juices. Hydrochloric acid activates the intrinsic factor in the stomach that is necessary for the absorption of vitamin B12 (see pages 55 and 56). It also helps prevent bacterial overgrowth in the stomach and intestines.

NOTES ON DEFICIENCY

Chloride deficiency is very rare, but it can occur in situations of heavy fluid loss, such as diarrhea, vomiting, heavy sweating, and diuretic use.

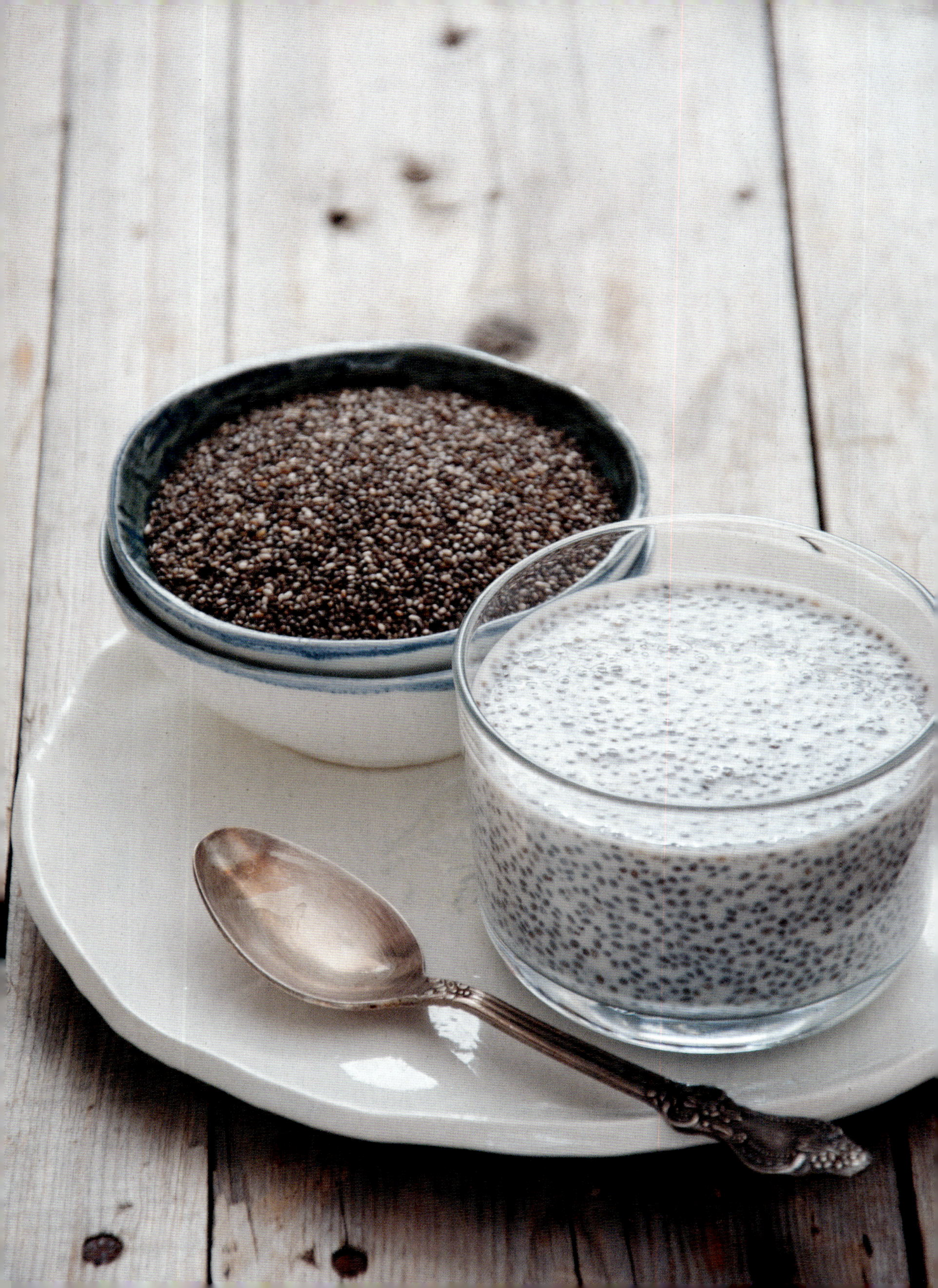

[MAGNESIUM]

THE **CALMING** MINERAL

RECOMMENDED DIETARY ALLOWANCE (RDA)

Men (19–30 years)	400 mg
Women (19–30 years)	310 mg
Men (31+ years)	420 mg
Women (31+ years)	320 mg
Pregnancy (14–18 years)	400 mg
Lactation (14–18 years)	360 mg
Pregnancy (19–30 years)	350 mg
Lactation (19–30 years)	310 mg
Pregnancy (31–50 years)	360 mg
Lactation (31–50 years)	320 mg

Magnesium, sometimes referred to as the "original chill pill," has been gaining attention in recent years for its possible role in lifting mood.

GOOD ALL-ROUNDER

While the impact of magnesium in mental health and disease prevention continues to be explored, it's well known that this essential mineral is involved in more than 300 enzyme reactions in the body. You may also recognize it as a common ingredient in medications, including the laxative Milk of Magnesia and various medicines for treating heartburn. The applications of this mineral really do seem endless!

Magnesium is abundant in the diet and can be found in several plant and animal foods. Still, almost half of Americans of all ages do not meet the RDA. Some experts believe that chronically low magnesium intake contributes to the development of common diseases that affect the US population, including heart disease and type 2 diabetes.

COMMON FOOD SOURCES

Leafy green vegetables are rich sources of magnesium, since the mineral makes up part of the chlorophyll in these plants. Whole grains are also considered good sources of this nutrient, but refined grains that have the nutrient-rich bran removed contain less magnesium. An ounce of pumpkin seeds and a cup each of brown rice and black beans, all mixed together, provide about enough magnesium to meet daily needs.

Pumpkin seeds (1 oz, roasted)	156 mg
Black beans (1 cup, cooked)	120 mg
Chia seeds (1 oz)	111 mg
Navy beans (1 cup, cooked)	96 mg
Brown rice (1 cup, cooked)	86 mg
Mackerel (3 oz, cooked)	82 mg
Almonds (1 oz, roasted)	80 mg
Spinach (½ cup, cooked)	78 mg
Dark chocolate (70–85%, 1 oz)	65 mg
Peanuts (1 oz, raw)	48 mg
Blackstrap molasses (1 tbsp)	48 mg
Plain yogurt (1 cup, low-fat)	42 mg
Beets (1 cup, raw)	31 mg

ROLE IN THE BODY

In the body, magnesium participates in more than 300 metabolic reactions, including fat and carbohydrate metabolism and DNA and RNA synthesis. Magnesium also helps potassium and calcium get transported across cell membranes, therefore assisting in muscle contraction and heart rhythm.

Due to its importance in bodily functions, magnesium is a nutrient of interest in disease prevention and treatment. Studies have found inverse relationships between magnesium intake and high blood pressure, atherosclerosis, insulin resistance, osteoporosis, migraines, major depression, and anxiety. However, the extent to which magnesium supplements may help reduce the risk of developing these diseases is unclear.

USING SUPPLEMENTS

Even though many Americans may have insufficient magnesium intake, increasing intake through diet instead of supplements should be the first step. Adverse effects of excess magnesium consumption from supplements (but not foods) include diarrhea, low blood pressure, confusion, lethargy, and muscle weakness. Individuals with impaired kidney function are at increased risk of toxicity. The UL for magnesium from supplements is set at 350 mg per day.

DID YOU KNOW?

While dietary fiber can decrease the absorption of magnesium in the body, this is not a concern if your diet includes plenty of magnesium-rich foods.

NOTES ON DEFICIENCY

Overt magnesium deficiency is rare, mainly because the kidneys can preserve magnesium in the body by limiting excretion. Individuals with chronic alcoholism or excessive magnesium loss due to health conditions or the use of some medications may be at risk of deficiency. Symptoms include loss of appetite, fatigue, nausea, and eventually low blood calcium or potassium in severe cases.

Inadequate intake

Inadequate dietary magnesium intake is more common than true deficiency and may affect 48% of Americans. This may be more likely in certain populations, including older adults and individuals with GI diseases or type 2 diabetes who do not consume enough magnesium and/or have impaired magnesium absorption. Habitually low intake of magnesium may be linked to disease development, but the effects are still not fully understood.

MINERAL TIPS

Magnesium levels drop during menstruation, so eating magnesium-rich foods may help ease pain, fatigue, and cramping. One such food is dark chocolate. Experts also suggest that chocolate boosts low energy resulting from hormonal changes. So, whether it's helpful because of the magnesium or the energy boost, dark chocolate made with 70% or more cocoa and little added sugar can be a nutritious snack for menstruating women.

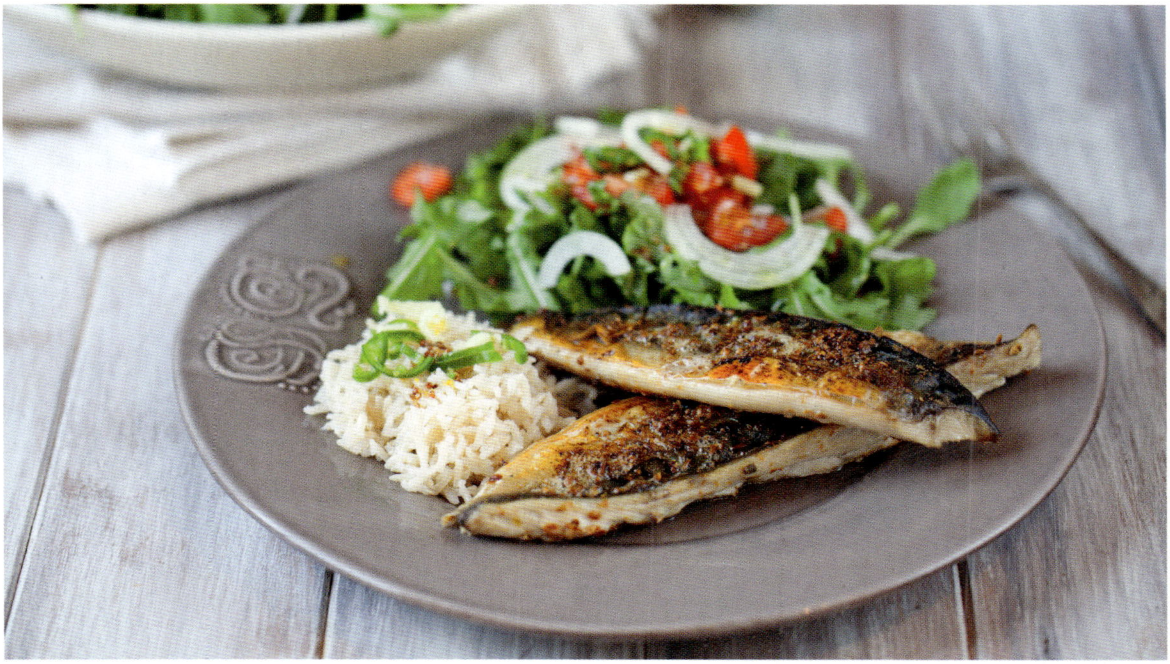

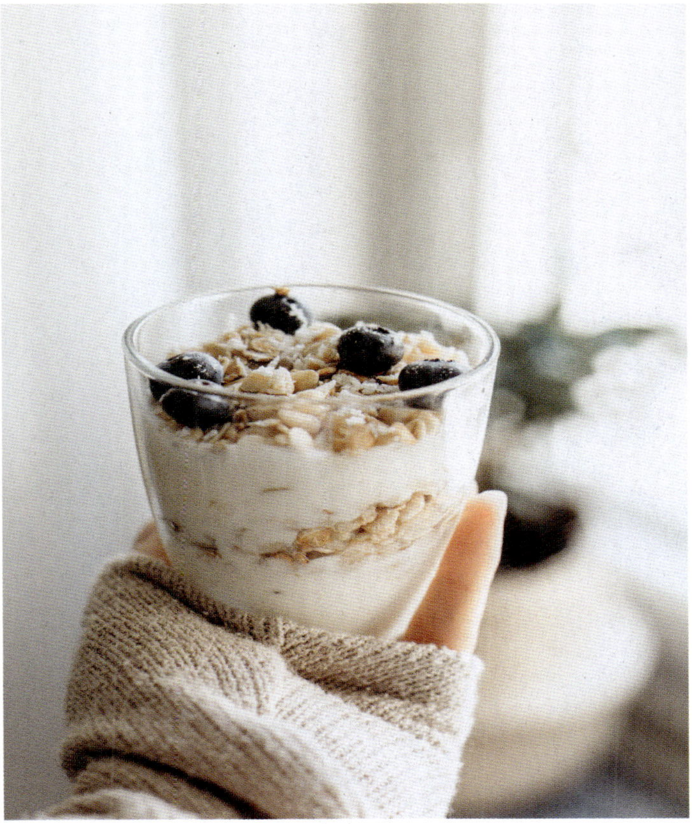

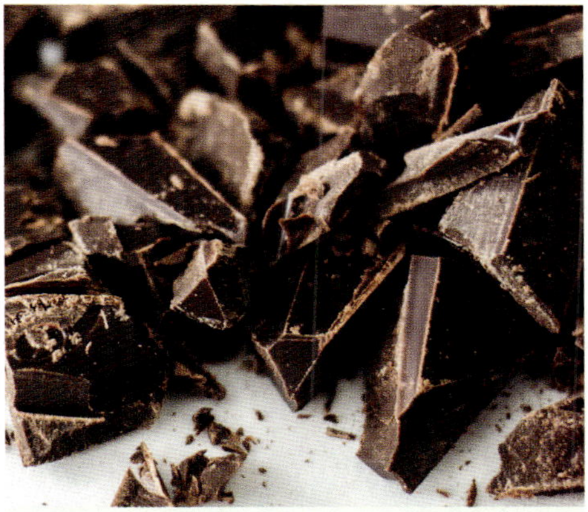

IN THE KITCHEN

CHOCOLATE BARK

Melt 12 oz dark chocolate in the microwave, stirring at 30-second intervals. Spread onto a baking sheet lined with parchment paper. Sprinkle with 1/4 cup each chopped pistachios, almonds, and dried apricots. Chill until hardened (30 mins). Break into pieces and sprinkle with flaky sea salt.

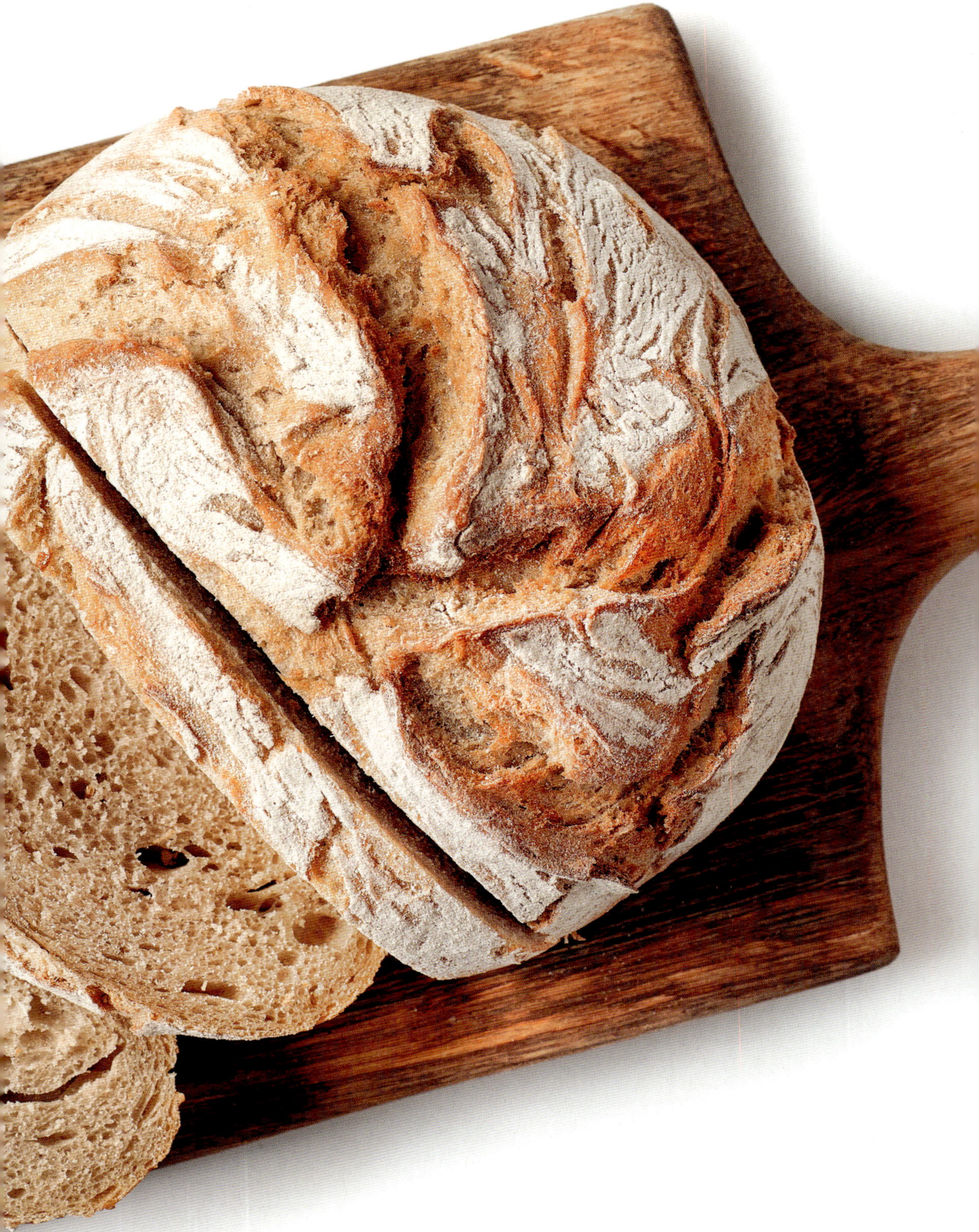

[PHOSPHORUS]

THE **CELL MEMBRANE** BUILDER

RECOMMENDED DIETARY ALLOWANCE (RDA)

Men and women	700 mg
Pregnancy and lactation (14–18 years)	1,250 mg
Pregnancy and lactation (19+ years)	700 mg

If you regularly read food labels, you have probably come across phosphorus in more foods than you might have expected.

ADDITIVE NUTRIENT

Phosphorus is a component of food additives, including phosphoric acid, sodium phosphate, or sodium polyphosphate, found in many canned and bottled drinks, processed meats, and ready-to-eat foods. The mineral also exists naturally in meat and dairy products, as well as in an abundance of fruits, vegetables, and other plant foods.

In the body, this major mineral is mostly found in bones and teeth, but it impacts many different systems and processes. In addition to providing structure to cell membranes, phosphorus influences gene transcription and energy metabolism.

Most Americans get more than enough phosphorus from their diets. Intake may even be higher than estimated, since many population-based studies do not account for phosphorus coming from additives. High phosphorus intakes may be related to increased risk of heart and bone diseases, although research on the health risks of excessive phosphorus is mixed.

COMMON FOOD SOURCES

The best sources of naturally occurring phosphorus include dairy products, fish, and meats, but it also exists in plant-based foods. A cup of milk, a serving of chicken, and a couple ounces of cashews provide enough phosphorus for one day.

Plain yogurt (8 oz, nonfat)	306 mg
2% milk (1 cup)	226 mg
Atlantic salmon (3 oz, cooked)	214 mg
Mozzarella cheese (1.5 oz)	197 mg
Chicken breast (3 oz, roasted)	182 mg
Lentils (½ cup, boiled)	178 mg
Cashew nuts (1 oz, roasted)	139 mg
Russet potato (1 medium, baked)	123 mg
Green peas (½ cup, boiled)	94 mg
Corn tortilla (1 medium)	82 mg
Whole wheat bread (1 slice)	68 mg
Carbonated cola drink (12 oz)	41 mg
Apple (1 medium)	20 mg

ROLE IN THE BODY

In the forms of hydroxyapatite and phospholipids, phosphorus provides structure to bones and cell membranes, respectively. About 85% of phosphorus in the body can be found in the bones and teeth, whereas 15% of the mineral exists in the blood and tissues.

Phosphorus is also part of adenosine triphosphate (ATP), the energy-carrying molecule found in all cells, as well as DNA and RNA, which store and transmit genetic information. The mineral serves as a buffer in the body, helping to maintain acid-base balance and normal pH.

NOTES ON DEFICIENCY

Since dietary intake generally meets or exceeds the RDA in the United States, phosphorus deficiency is very rare. Individuals with certain genetic disorders or severe malnutrition are at increased risk of deficiency, characterized by wasting, bone pain, confusion, and a higher susceptibility to infections.

USING SUPPLEMENTS

Phosphorus is widely available in the food supply, making supplements unnecessary. In fact, most people get too much dietary phosphorus. The UL for total phosphorus intake from food and supplements is 4,000 mg for adults ages 19–70 years and lactating women, 3,000 mg for adults 71 years of age and older, and 3,500 mg for pregnant women.

DID YOU KNOW?

The phosphorus in nuts, seeds, and grains is about 50% less available for use in the body than phosphorus from other sources.

MINERAL TIPS

Some plant-based foods contain phosphorus, in a form known as phytic acid or phytate. Since the human digestive system cannot break phosphorus away from phytate, the phosphorus from beans, peas, cereals, and seeds is not well absorbed.

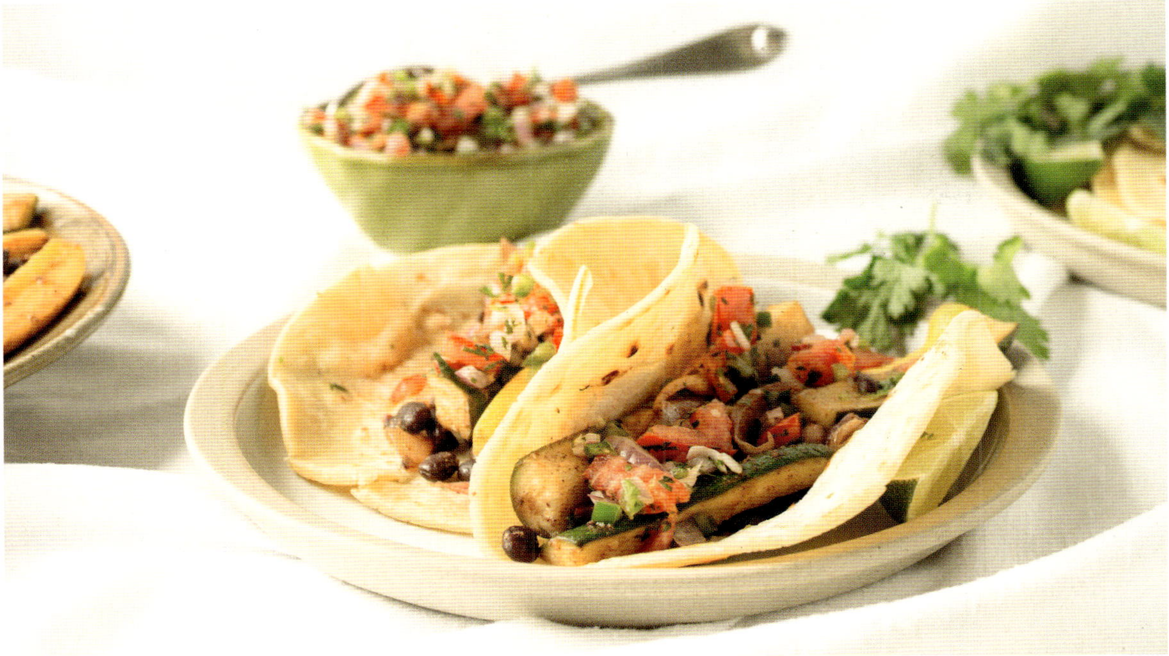

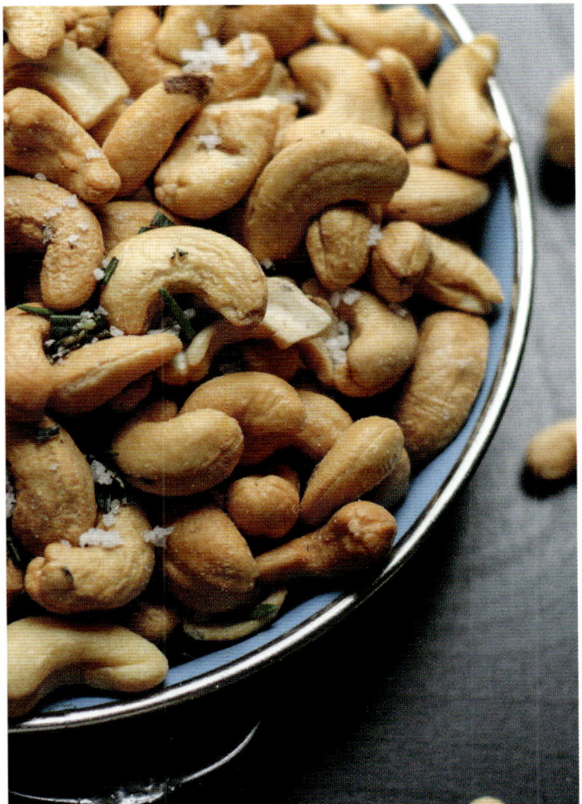

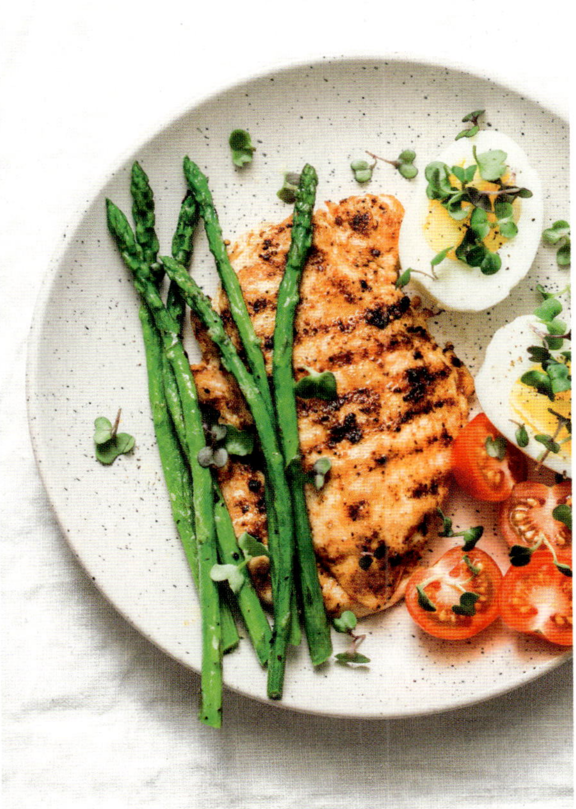

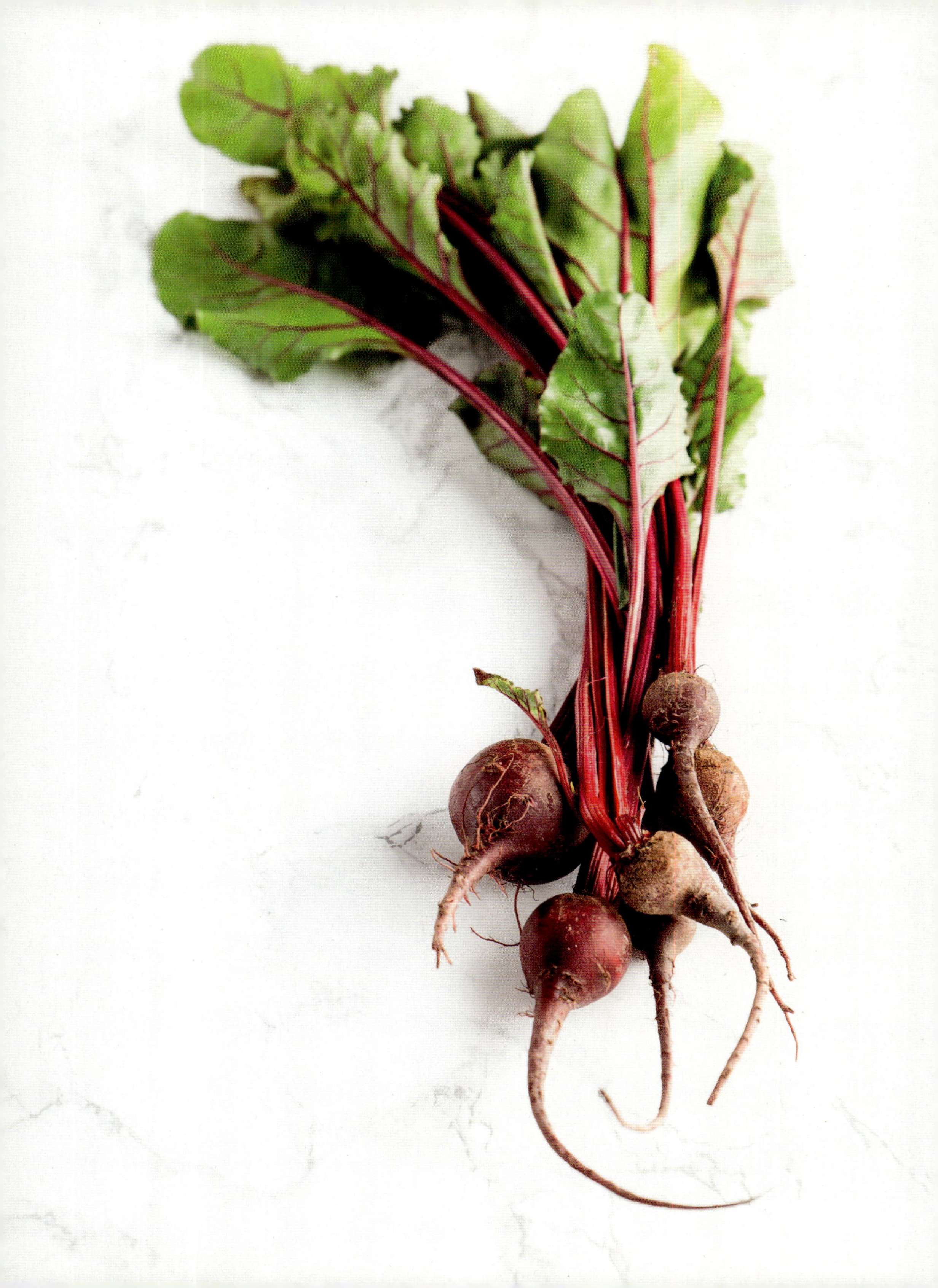

[POTASSIUM]

– THE **BLOOD PRESSURE** MINERAL –

ADEQUATE INTAKE (AI)

Men	3,400 mg
Women	2,600 mg
Pregnancy (14–18 years)	2,600 mg
Lactation (14–18 years)	2,500 mg
Pregnancy (19–50 years)	2,900 mg
Lactation (19–50 years)	2,800 mg

Potassium and bananas are grouped together like calcium and milk—over the years you've probably been told to eat bananas to increase your intake of this mineral. But do you know much else about it?

GREAT REGULATOR

As a major electrolyte in the body, potassium works closely with sodium to maintain fluid volume. These two minerals also regulate blood pressure, and low potassium intake coupled with high sodium intake may contribute to hypertension. In fact, the 2015–2020 Dietary Guidelines for Americans identified potassium as a "nutrient of public health concern" and it is now featured on food labels. Americans generally do not meet the AI levels for potassium, and at the same time, get too much sodium.

COMMON FOOD SOURCES

In a diet that includes plenty of fruits and vegetables, potassium is abundant. A banana at breakfast, a cup of lentils with lunch, a serving of dried apricots for a snack, and a baked potato with dinner would provide enough potassium to meet daily needs. Most salt substitutes also contain potassium chloride as a replacement for sodium chloride.

Dried apricots (½ cup)	1,101 mg
Potato (1 medium, baked, with skin)	926 mg
Lentils (1 cup, cooked)	731 mg
Avocado (1 cup, sliced)	708 mg
Acorn squash (1 cup, mashed)	644 mg
Kidney beans (1 cup, canned)	607 mg
Beets (1 cup, cooked slices)	518 mg
Banana (1 medium)	422 mg
Artichoke (1 medium, cooked)	343 mg
Spinach (2 cups, raw)	334 mg
Chicken breast (3 oz, grilled)	332 mg
Tomato (1 medium, raw)	292 mg
Pistachios (1 oz, raw)	285 mg
Cantaloupe (½ cup, cubed)	214 mg
Cucumber (1 cup, sliced)	152 mg
Coffee (1 cup, brewed)	116 mg
Cilantro (½ cup)	21 mg

ROLE IN THE BODY

Potassium is the main positively charged ion in intracellular fluid. Both potassium and sodium exist in different concentrations inside and outside cells, and these differences create an important activity known as the cell membrane potential. The cell membrane potential is tightly controlled and plays a vital role in nerve impulse transmission and muscle contraction.

The interconnectedness between the two minerals potassium and sodium is also the underlying reason for potassium's role in blood pressure. Research suggests that increasing potassium intake can help lower blood pressure, in part by increasing the excretion of sodium in the urine. Potassium also promotes vasodilation, meaning it helps blood vessels open and relax.

USING SUPPLEMENTS

Multivitamin-mineral supplements only contain 99 mg (or less) of potassium, since the FDA has imposed regulations on how much potassium some products can have. This is mostly because drugs that contain potassium chloride in amounts higher than 99 mg have been linked to small bowel lesions. The best way to increase potassium consumption is through diet.

NOTES ON DEFICIENCY

Potassium deficiency, marked by fatigue, muscle weakness, breathing issues, and cardiac arrhythmias, is rare but can occur in individuals using diuretics or who have severe potassium losses due to diarrhea or vomiting.

Inadequate intake

If potassium consumption falls short of the adequate intake but is enough to prevent deficiency, it's referred to as potassium inadequacy. Individuals with inflammatory bowel disease or frequent diuretic and laxative use may be at high risk of inadequacy.

HIGH BLOOD POTASSIUM

Individuals with advanced chronic kidney disease may be at risk of hyperkalemia (high blood potassium), since impaired kidney function makes it more difficult to excrete potassium in the urine. It's beneficial to speak with a registered dietitian or physician about appropriate potassium intake if you have kidney disease.

DID YOU KNOW?

Not getting enough potassium can increase sensitivity to salt, which means that sodium intake will affect blood pressure more than usual.

MINERAL TIPS

Besides being a source of potassium, coffee contains many beneficial compounds. In fact, it is the number one source of antioxidants in the American diet (see Antioxidants, pages 140–41). It is best drunk black or with moderate amounts of milk/cream.

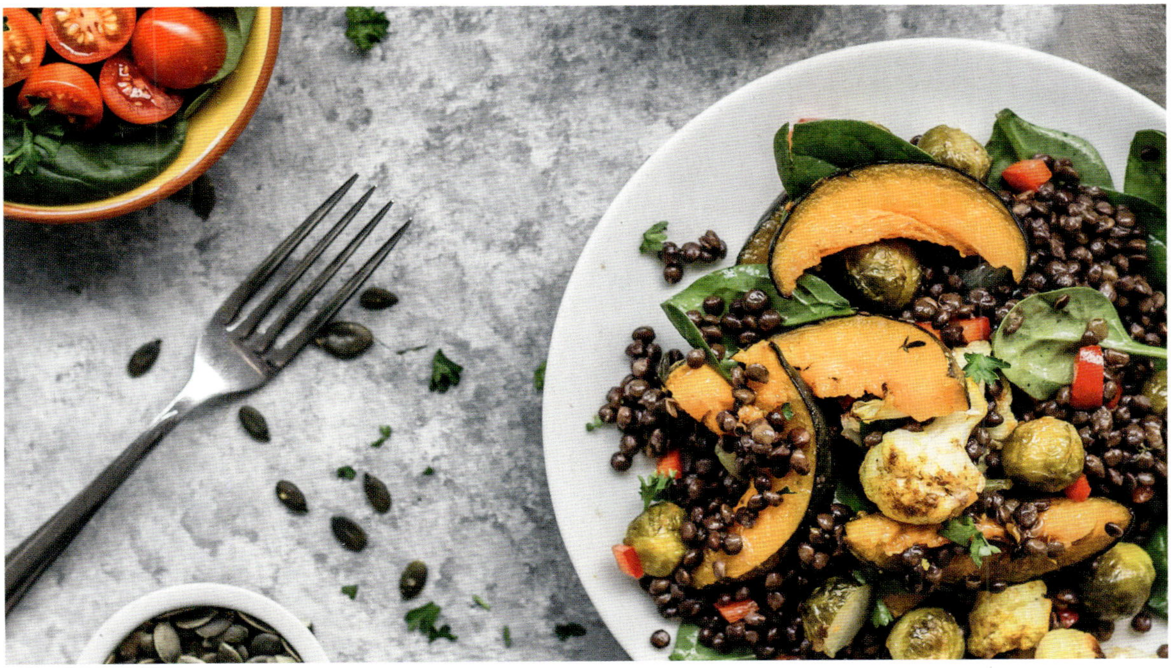

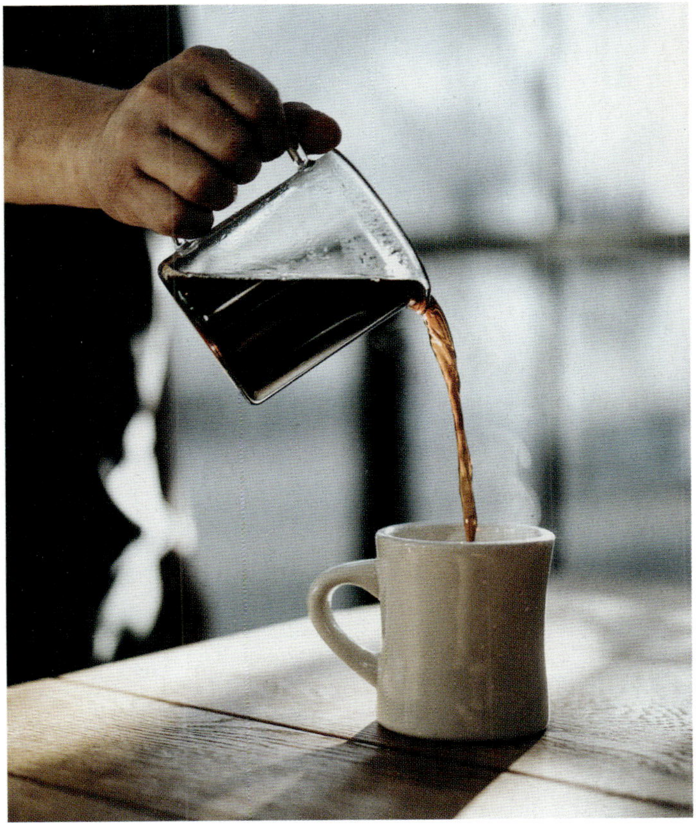

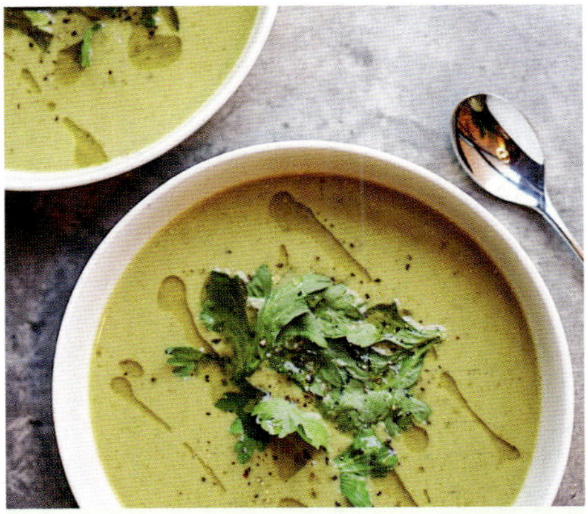

IN THE KITCHEN

WHOLESOME SOUP

For a delicious meal that's loaded with potassium, blend a lentil soup just before serving and top with a handful of cilantro leaves.

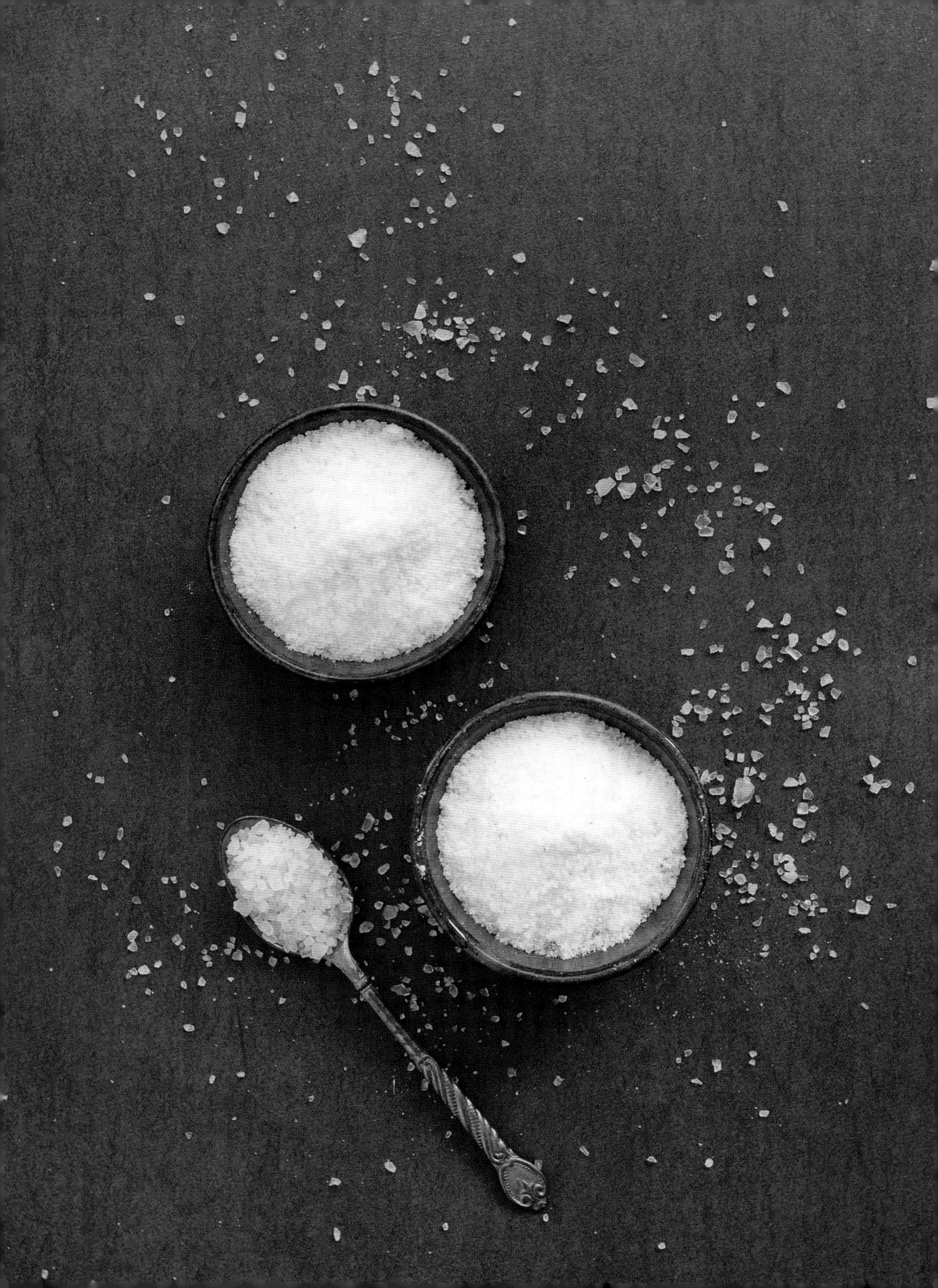

[SODIUM]

ADEQUATE INTAKE (AI)

Men and women	1,500 mg
Pregnancy and lactation	1,500 mg

THE **FLAVOR** ENHANCER

Salt is one of the most versatile and beloved cooking ingredients. It adds flavor to dishes and helps preserve foods. But when it comes to salt intake, it's easy to have too much of a good thing.

BENEFICIAL INTAKE

Sodium works with the other electrolytes to maintain blood pressure and plays a pivotal role in the body's water balance systems. Even though it has many important functions, high dietary sodium intake is a problem and can lead to high blood pressure and other health issues.

To reduce the risk of hypertension and heart disease, the National Academy of Medicine recommends that adults keep their daily sodium intakes to 2,300 mg or less. This amount was also the recommended AI until 2019, when the National Academy of Medicine revised the AI for sodium to 1,500 mg. The change reflects the abundance of evidence suggesting that sodium intakes below 2,300 mg have potential long-term health benefits adults. See page 92 for ways in which you can reduce your sodium intake to beneficial levels.

HIGH-SODIUM FOODS

The biggest source of sodium in the diet is salt added during food processing, followed by salt added at the table and in cooking. Few foods contain naturally occurring sodium. Below are some examples of high sodium foods.
A diet rich in fruits, vegetables, and whole grains will be much lower in sodium than one that includes many of the foods on this list.

Salted potato chips (8-oz bag)	1,196 mg
Ham (3 oz, minced)	1,059 mg
Macaroni & cheese (1 cup, boxed)	869 mg
Chicken noodle soup (1 cup, canned)	789 mg
Cheese spread (1 oz, pasteurized)	416 mg
Beef hot dog (1)	409 mg
Dill pickle (1 spear)	283 mg

USING SUPPLEMENTS

The average sodium intake in the United States far exceeds the AI. Supplements or "salt pills" should not be used unless there is a specific reason for taking them.

ROLE IN THE BODY

Sodium levels in the body are regulated by the kidneys and dictate water balance. When dietary intake of sodium is high, thirst increases and the body holds on to water to achieve the proper blood levels of sodium. This raises blood volume and blood pressure. With a decreased intake of sodium, the kidneys do not retain as much water, again to maintain the proper sodium levels. These mechanisms are why excess sodium consumption can lead to high blood pressure, the main preventable risk factor for heart disease.

NOTES ON DEFICIENCY

In rare instances, not getting enough sodium from foods can cause low blood sodium levels, known as hyponatremia. Marked by headaches, vomiting, cramping, fatigue, and even brain swelling or coma, this condition more often occurs in hospitalized patients or those with hypertension, diabetes, stroke, cancer, or extremely high water consumption.

MINERAL TIPS

The new sodium AI of 1,500 mg equates to 3,800 mg of salt, or just ⅔ teaspoon! Check labels for the sodium contents of the foods you are eating. If you are watching your sodium intake, look for low, reduced-sodium, and "no salt added" versions of canned vegetables, beans, and condiments.

DID YOU KNOW?

Draining and rinsing canned veggies and beans may reduce sodium content by as much as 40%.

LOWERING YOUR SODIUM INTAKE

High dietary sodium intake is concerning, since it may increase the chances of developing hypertension. About one in three American adults has high blood pressure, and prevalence is highest among Black men and women. Dietary changes can help you cut back on sodium, which may reduce the risk of getting hypertension and help with disease management. Here are some tips for low-sodium cooking:

Go natural: Replace foods that have been processed or preserved with salt with natural alternatives—fresh and frozen fruits and vegetables, whole grains, healthy fats such as olive oil and avocado, eggs, and lean meats.

Skip the salt shaker: Numerous pantry staples will provide flavor without the need for adding sodium. Try lemon juice, vinegars, cayenne pepper, chili powder, rosemary, garlic, dried onion, ginger, and cinnamon in place of salt.

Do-it-yourself: Two of the biggest sources of sodium, canned soups and beans, are very easy to make from scratch. Look for recipes that use bay leaves or other herbs and spices in addition to or in lieu of salt.

Check the label: When buying ready-to-eat meals, choose options that have less than 500–600 mg sodium per serving—around one-third of the daily AI.

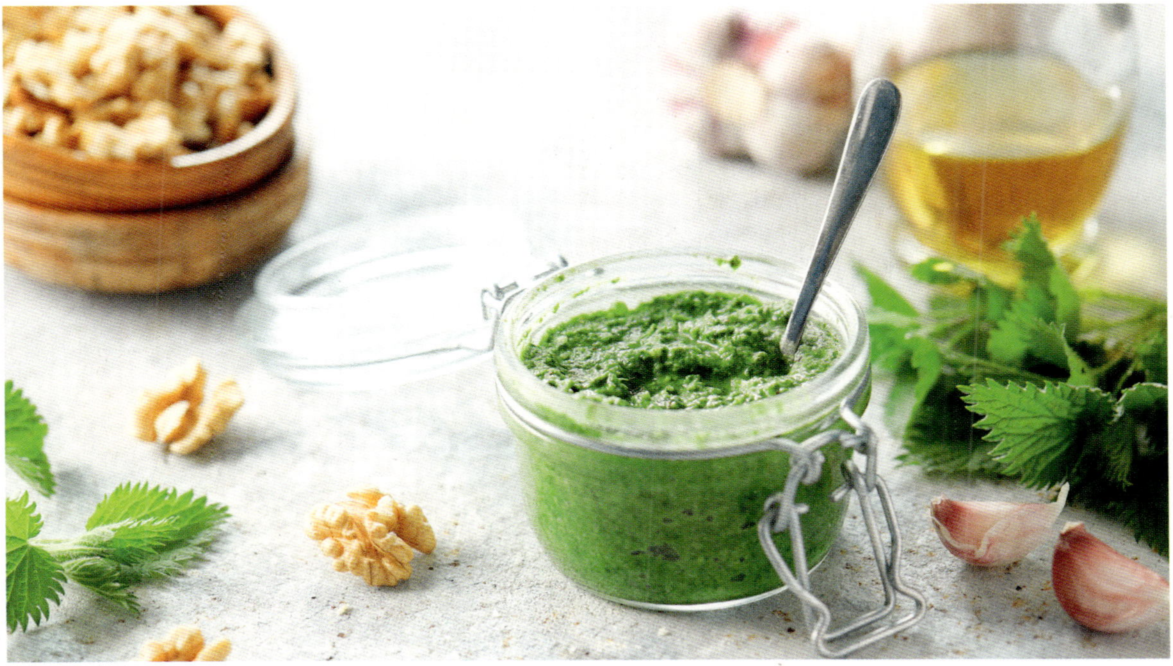

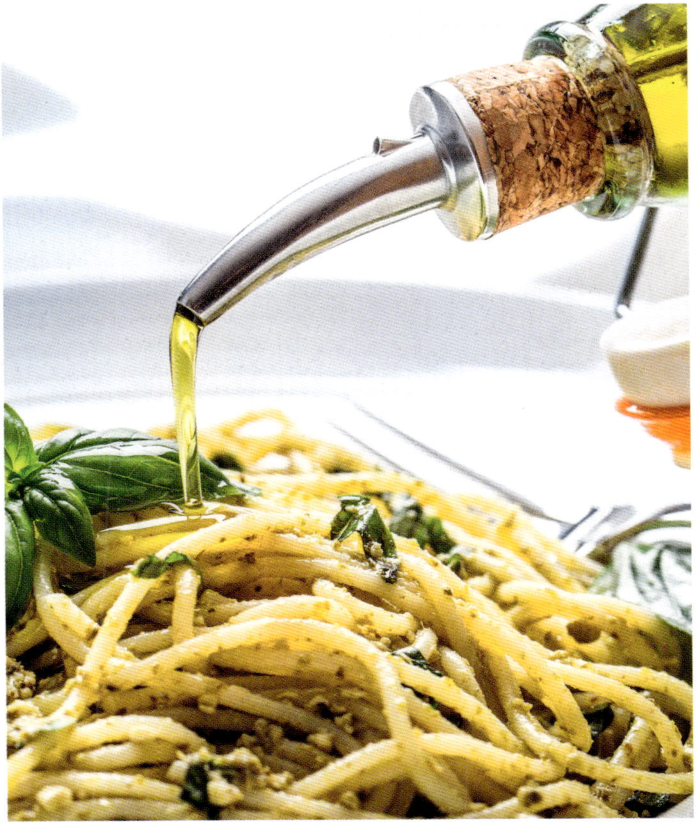

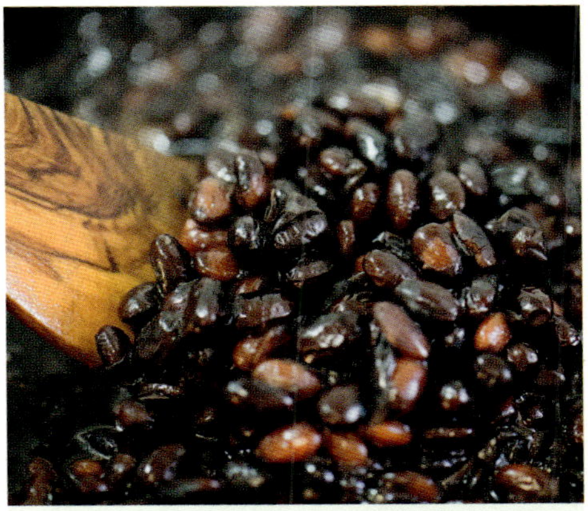

IN THE KITCHEN

DIY BLACK BEANS

Soak 1 cup dried black beans overnight in 8 cups water. Drain, rinse, and discard any shriveled or broken beans. Bring the soaked beans to a boil in a large pot with 4 cups water, 1/2 tsp salt, 1 bay leaf, and 3 cloves smashed garlic. Cover, and simmer for 45–60 minutes, until tender. Remove bay leaf before adding to soups and salads.

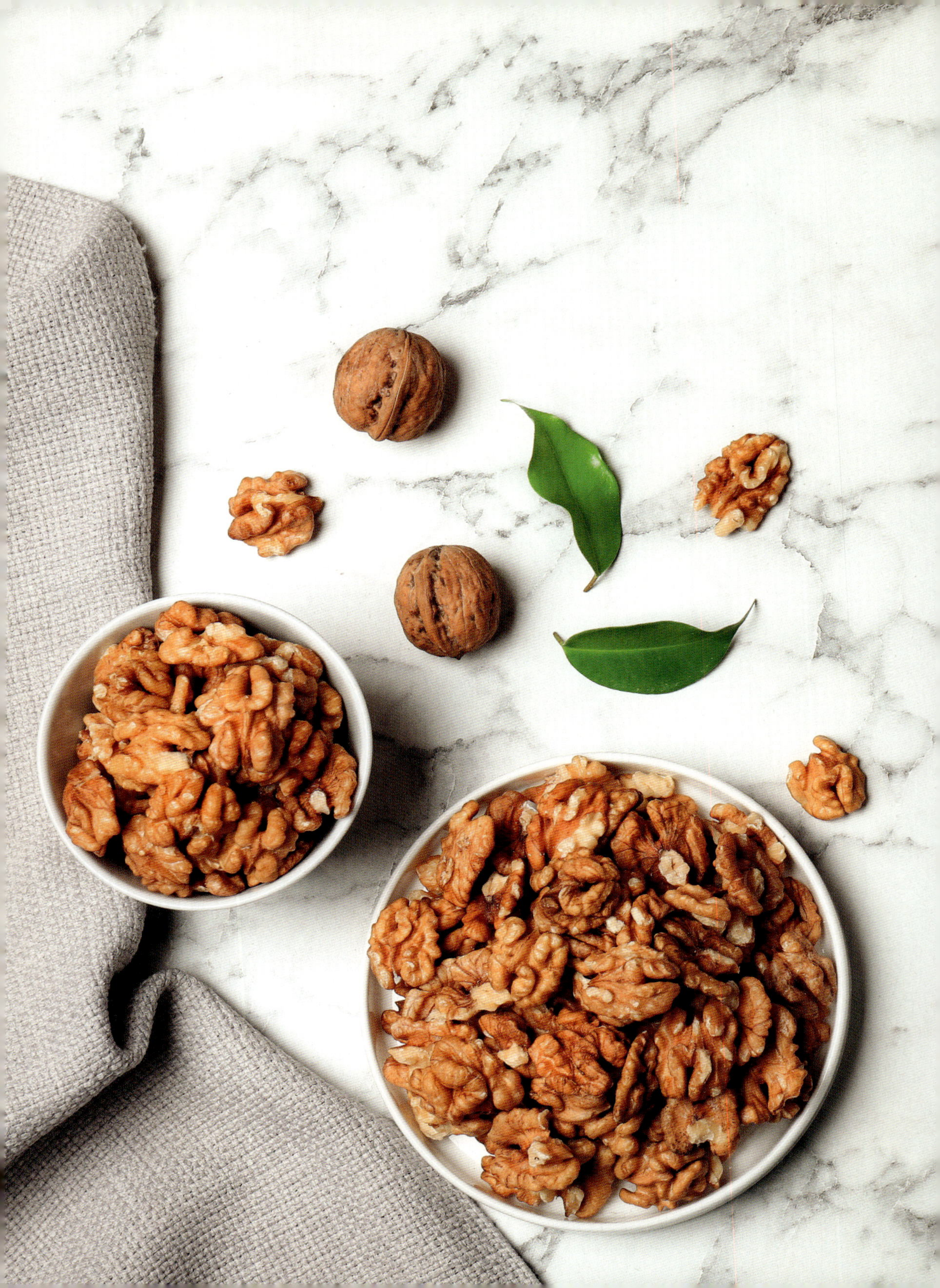

[SULFUR]

THE **PROTEIN** BRIDGE

RECOMMENDED DIETARY ALLOWANCE (RDA)

There is no RDA for sulfur, since it's assumed that most people meet their needs through protein intake.

Sulfur does not stand alone as a nutrient, but mainly exists as part of the amino acids methionine and cysteine. Therefore, protein-rich foods are the best sources of sulfur in the diet. Primary functions in the body relate to protein folding and structure, but sulfur has other roles.

COMMON FOOD SOURCES

Animal proteins, including, chicken, turkey, beef, ham, eggs, cheese, fish, and seafood, all provide sulfur. Plant-based sources include soybeans, white beans, walnuts, almonds, dried apricots, oats, and pearl barley. Sulfur is also found in some vegetables.

USING SUPPLEMENTS

Sulfur is mainly found as dimethyl sulfoxide (DMSO) and methylsulfonylmethane (MSM) in supplements. MSM is sometimes used for joint pain and arthritis, and placebo-controlled trials suggest that it's effective for these issues. A healthy adult with a varied diet does not need sulfur supplements. Some supplemental forms of sulfur, especially DMSO, can be dangerous and cause unwanted side effects. Speak with a health care provider before taking supplements of any kind.

ROLE IN THE BODY

Sulfur is a key component of disulfide bridges, which come together when proteins fold. The shapes of proteins dictate what they do, and so sulfur is vital to protein function. The mineral also assists in reactions involved in the body's defenses against oxidative damage, specifically the production of the antioxidant glutathione.

NOTES ON DEFICIENCY

Sulfur deficiency has not been seen in humans, and sulfur intake is considered adequate in those who consume enough protein for their needs.

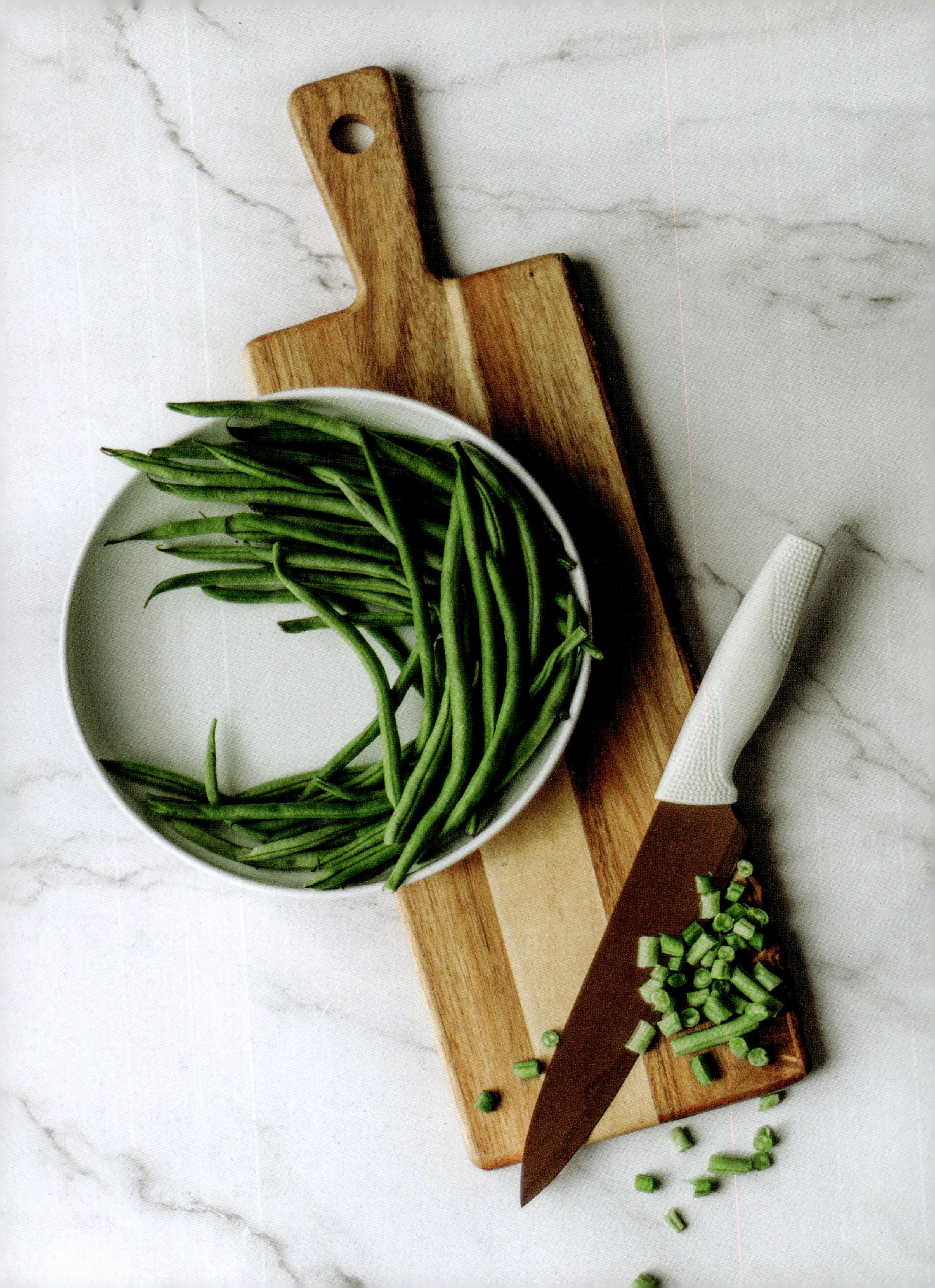

[CHROMIUM]

THE **INSULIN** ACTIVATOR

ADEQUATE INTAKE (AI)

Men (19–50 years)	35 mcg
Women (19–50 years)	25 mcg
Men (51+ years)	30 mcg
Women (51+ years)	20 mcg
Pregnancy (14–18 years)	29 mcg
Lactation (14–18 years)	44 mcg
Pregnancy (19–50 years)	30 mcg
Lactation (19–50 years)	45 mcg

Health gurus and the diet industry may try to convince you otherwise, but there are still many unknowns when it comes to nutrition. And the history of chromium is just one example of the evolving nutritional knowledge base.

AIDING INSULIN ACTION

In 2001, experts classified chromium as an essential nutrient, but recent research suggests that an absence of chromium does not actually inhibit proper bodily functioning. In the United States, the status of chromium has not been revisited since that time, but European experts stated that chromium is not an essential nutrient based on current evidence in 2014.

Despite these ongoing debates, it's clear that chromium does have important functions. As a vital nutrient for insulin action, this trace mineral may be especially important for the American population, of which over 30 million people have type 2 diabetes.

COMMON FOOD SOURCES

While many foods provide chromium, the amount each contains largely depends on soil conditions and manufacturing processes. As such, it is difficult to get an accurate measurement, so the values below should be viewed as estimated, rather than definitive, amounts. Eating a cup of broccoli, an English muffin, and a glass of tomato juice throughout the day would provide about enough chromium to meet your needs.

Broccoli (1 cup, raw)	22 mcg
Grape juice (1 cup)	7.5 mcg
English muffin (1, whole wheat)	3.6 mcg
Brewer's yeast (1 tbsp)	3.3 mcg
Green beans (1 cup, raw)	2.2 mcg
Turkey breast (3 oz, cooked)	1.7 mcg
Tomato juice (1 cup)	1.5 mcg
Banana (1 medium)	1.0 mcg
Orange (1 medium)	0.4 mcg

ROLE IN THE BODY

Trivalent chromium, the main form of chromium in the body, is thought to be a cofactor for a molecule called chromodulin that enhances the action of insulin. When blood sugar increases, such as after a meal, insulin is the hormone that's released to bind to cells and help them take in glucose. Decreased insulin sensitivity can lead to high blood sugar levels and, eventually, type 2 diabetes.

Due to reasons that are not yet fully understood, chromium may improve insulin sensitivity. Some randomized controlled trials have found that chromium supplements may help lower fasting blood sugar concentrations in people with type 2 diabetes. However, other studies suggest that chromium supplementation is not effective in improving blood sugar control.

USING SUPPLEMENTS

Most people get enough chromium from food and don't need supplements, but they are sometimes used in the treatment of type 2 diabetes. There is no UL for chromium, but there may be concerns about the safety of long-term chromium supplementation.

DID YOU KNOW?

Stainless-steel food processing equipment, pots, and pans may transfer some chromium to food.

NOTES ON DEFICIENCY

Accurately detecting chromium status is difficult, so there isn't much information about deficiency. However, it is not thought to be common, and a balanced diet that includes a variety of food groups provides adequate chromium.

MINERAL TIPS

Diets high in simple sugars, including those from foods such as sugar-sweetened beverages, baked goods, and candy, may increase the excretion of chromium in the urine. Complex carbohydrates, such as whole grains, do not lead to as much chromium loss.

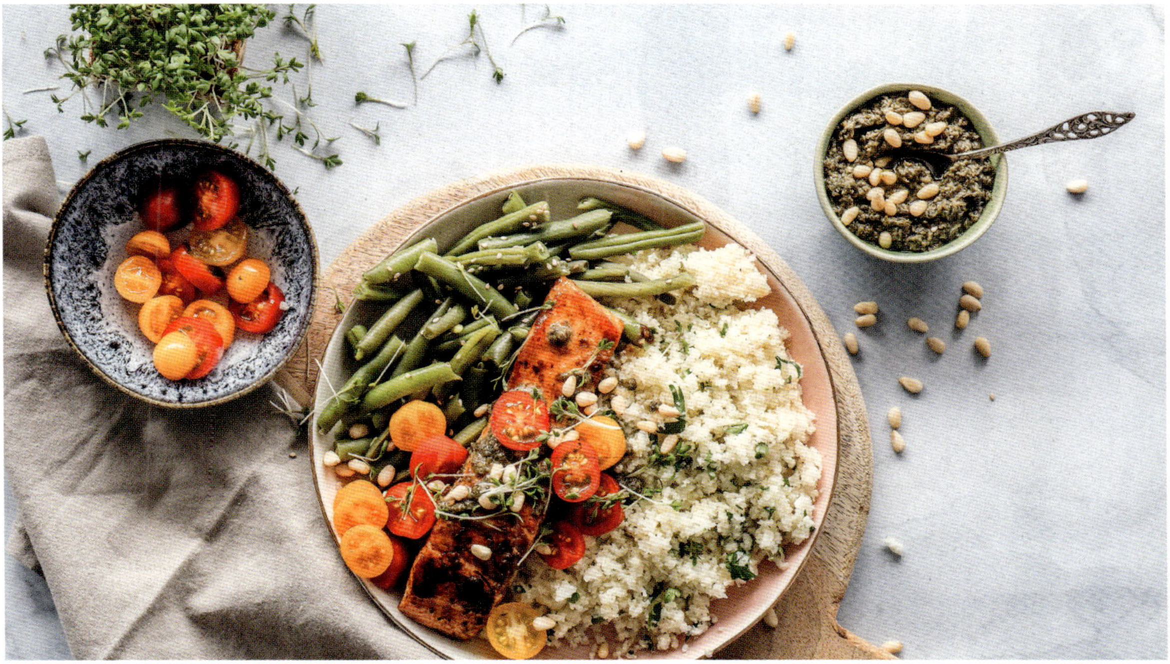

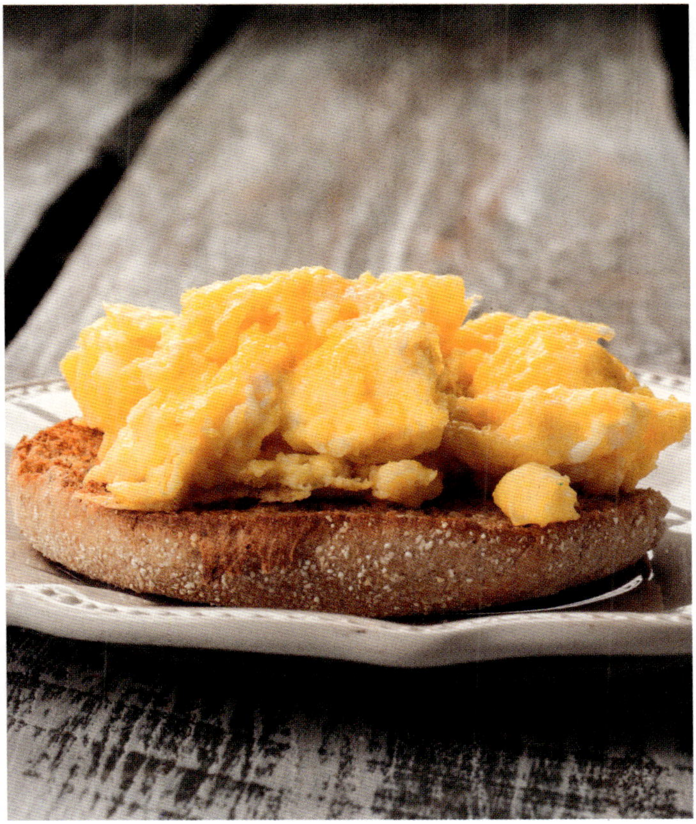

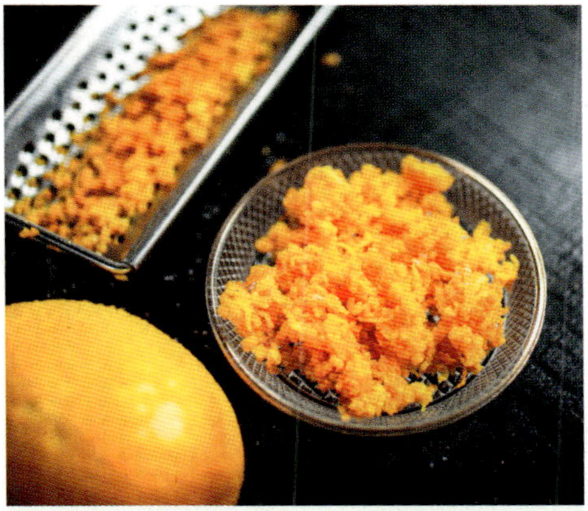

IN THE KITCHEN

ZINGY BROCCOLI

Vitamin C may increase chromium uptake. Try steamed broccoli with orange sauce for a side dish that provides both of these nutrients. To make the sauce, melt a couple tablespoons butter in a saucepan, then whisk in a few tablespoons orange juice and orange zest to taste.

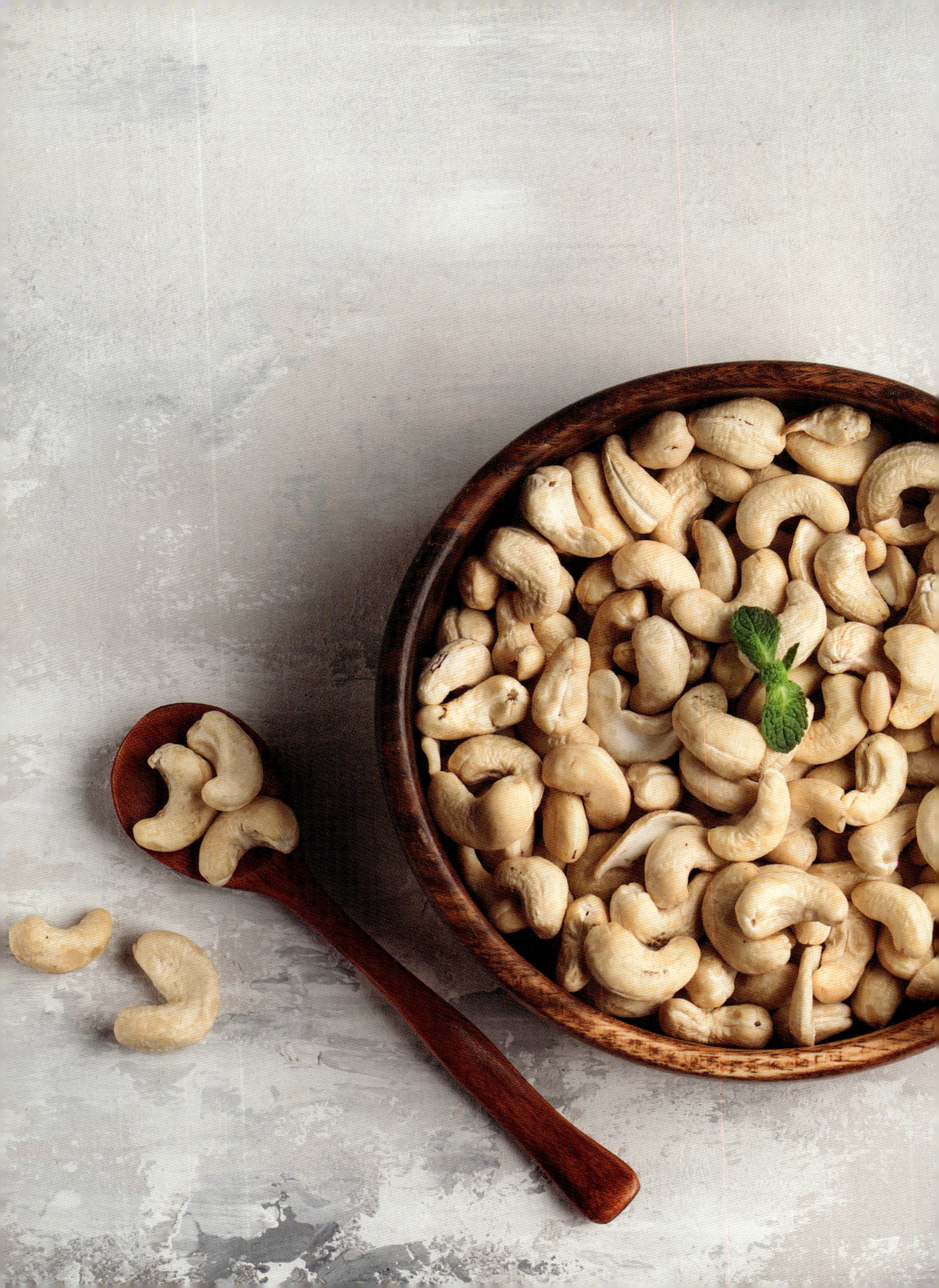

[COPPER]

RECOMMENDED DIETARY ALLOWANCE (RDA)

Men and women	900 mcg
Pregnancy and lactation	1,300 mcg

THE **PIGMENTATION** MINERAL

It may seem strange that copper, the mineral that provides the brown coating on pennies, is an essential nutrient for human health. But did you know that without copper, the body would not be able to perform iron metabolism, tissue formation, and many other processes?

Copper also supports immune function, bone mineralization, and brain health. Even though copper is needed in smaller amounts than major minerals, it's vital to get enough of this nutrient from foods. Shellfish provides significant amounts of copper, but there are plenty of plant-based sources for those who do not eat fish.

COMMON FOOD SOURCES

Shellfish and organ meats are some of the best sources of copper, and many plant foods also provide this nutrient. Just three ounces of cooked oysters contain enough copper for five days!

Eastern oysters (3 oz, cooked)	4,850 mcg
Potato (1 medium, cooked, flesh and skin)	675 mcg
Shiitake mushrooms (1/2 cup, cooked)	650 mcg
Cashew nuts (1 oz, roasted)	629 mcg
Sunflower seeds (1/4 cup, roasted)	615 mcg
Millet (1 cup, cooked)	280 mcg
Dried figs (1/2 cup)	214 mcg
Peanut butter (2 tbsp, chunky)	185 mcg
Ground turkey (3 oz, cooked)	128 mcg
Farina cereal (1 cup, hot, cooked with water)	104 mcg

ROLE IN THE BODY

Copper is part of several enzymes that play a role in energy production, as well as in the creation of connective tissue from collagen and elastin. The transport of iron from storage so that it can be used in the synthesis of red blood cells is also dependent on copper. For this reason, copper deficiency can lead to anemia or iron overload in the liver.

Since copper also plays a role in the normal functioning of the brain and nervous system, copper status may be connected to neurological conditions. For example, researchers are currently investigating a possible link between Alzheimer's disease and issues of copper metabolism. Finally, antioxidants known as superoxide dismutase (SOD) contain copper. SOD is found in red blood cells and most other cells as an important player in the body's antioxidant activity.

USING SUPPLEMENTS

Copper supplements are not usually necessary nor beneficial, since most adults meet or exceed copper intake from their diets. Excess copper intake over the long term may lead to liver damage. The UL for copper from food and supplements is 10 mg (10,000 mcg) per day.

DID YOU KNOW?

A copper-dependent enzyme is necessary for the creation of melanin, the pigment responsible for your skin's color.

NOTES ON DEFICIENCY

Copper deficiency, characterized by anemia, osteoporosis, and increased susceptibility to infection, is uncommon. Individuals with celiac, Crohn's, or Menkes disease may be at increased risk of copper inadequacy or deficiency.

MINERAL TIPS

Since zinc interferes with copper absorption, regular use of zinc supplements or zinc-containing creams can lead to copper deficiency. Taking high doses (50+ mg/day) of zinc supplements has been linked to decreased copper status.

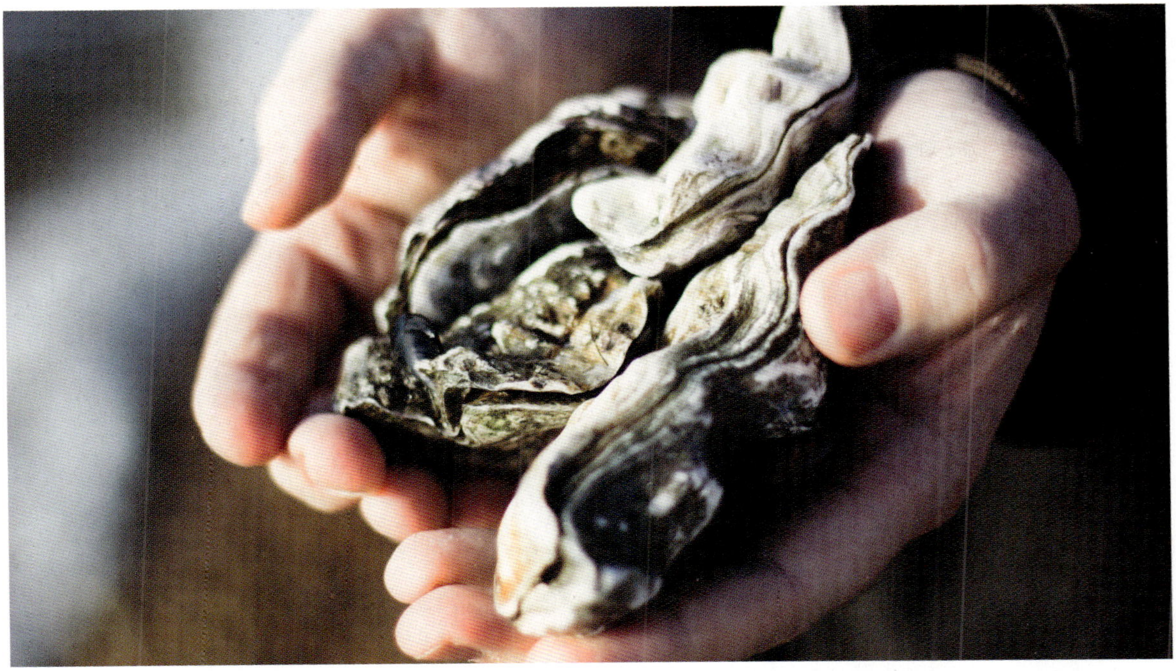

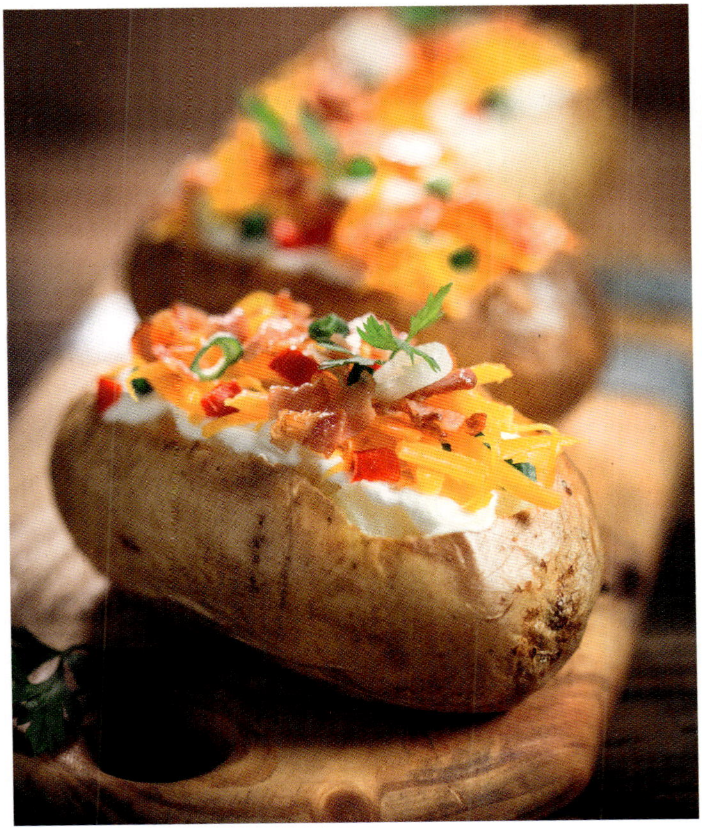

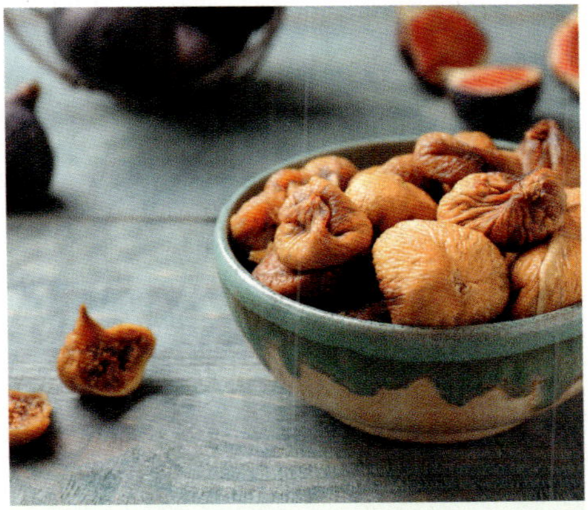

IN THE KITCHEN

FRUIT AND NUT FARINA

For a balanced breakfast that packs plenty of copper, try a bowl of farina cereal topped with ¼ cup each dried figs, roasted sunflower seeds, and roasted cashew nuts.

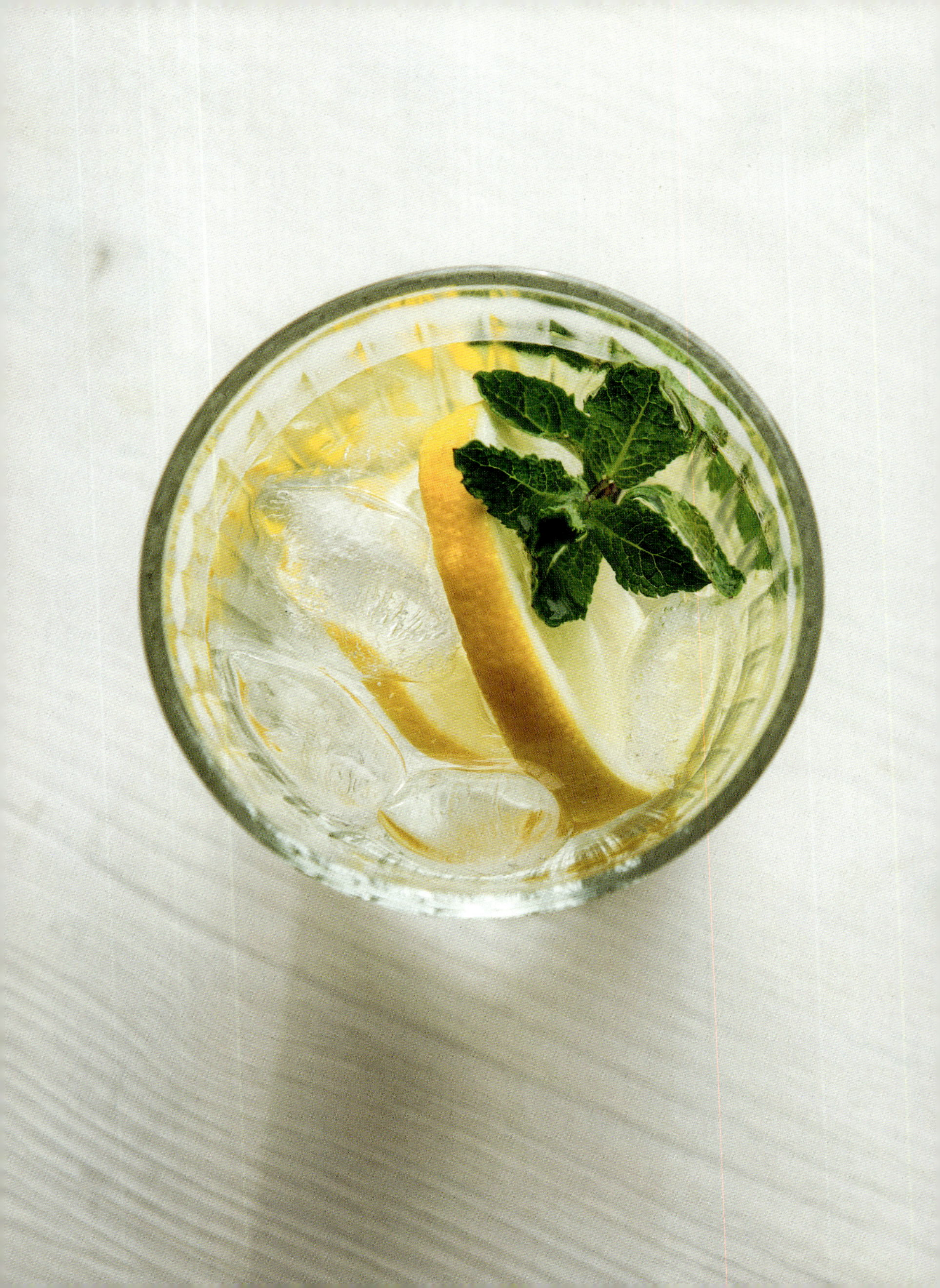

[FLUORIDE]

ADEQUATE INTAKE (AI)

Men	4 mg
Women	3 mg
Pregnancy and lactation	3 mg

THE **CAVITY** PREVENTER

If you're drinking a glass of water as you page through this book, then there's a good chance you're ingesting fluoride at the moment.

ALL ABOUT FLUORIDATION

To help prevent dental cavities, fluoride is added to community water systems in the United States. Drinking water is therefore the biggest source of fluoride in the food supply, but a few foods and beverages also contain this mineral. Some areas in Europe, Latin America, and Southeast Asia add fluoride to salt and milk, but these practices are not implemented in the United States.

While there have been some concerns that fluoride may increase the risk of chronic diseases, these claims are not backed by research. Instead, water fluoridation is largely considered safe and beneficial due to the positive effects on teeth.

COMMON FOOD SOURCES

Drinking fluoridated tap water is the best way to get fluoride. About 10 cups of water provide enough fluoride to meet daily needs. If you don't drink that much water or live in an area without fluoridated water, consider adding some of the following foods and beverages to your diet. Foods and drinks made with water, such as oatmeal, rice, and tea, will have varying amounts of fluoride depending on the fluoride content in the water. Dental products, including most toothpastes, mouth rinses, and gels applied by dentists, are also a source of fluoride. How much fluoride is ingested from these products depends on how much is swallowed.

Water (1 cup, fluoridated)	0.2–0.3 mg
Black tea (1 cup)	0.07–1.5 mg
Raisins (1/4 cup)	0.08 mg
Oatmeal (1/2 cup, cooked)	0.08 mg
Grapefruit juice (3/4 cup)	0.08 mg
Cottage cheese (1/2 cup)	0.04 mg
Rice (1/2 cup, cooked)	0.04 mg
Pork chop (3 oz, baked)	0.03 mg

ROLE IN THE BODY

Fluoride helps promote tooth mineralization and contributes to strong enamel, especially while teeth are developing. It also works to prevent tooth decay by stopping acid-producing bacteria from acting on teeth.

Some studies suggest that fluoride, in supplemental pharmacological doses but not in the amount found in fluoridated drinking water, may help prevent osteoporosis. However, these high doses come with serious side effects, including joint pain, calcium deficiency, and stress fractures.

NOTES ON DEFICIENCY

Fluoride deficiency is uncommon in the United States, and most people get enough from water and foods. The only known symptom of deficiency is increased risk of tooth decay.

USING SUPPLEMENTS

Fluoride supplementation should always be prescribed and monitored by a health care provider.

In areas without access to fluoridated drinking water, supplements may help reduce dental caries in children. Experts recommend 0.25–1 mg of supplements per day where water supplies contain 0–0.6 ppm (parts per million) fluoride. If you are concerned your child is not getting enough fluoride, speak with a pediatrician or dentist before starting supplements. It's unclear whether fluoride supplements help prevent cavity development in adults.

Getting too much fluoride in childhood when teeth are forming can lead to white flecks or stains on the teeth, a result of a condition known as dental fluorosis. Up to 41% of adolescents in the United States may have dental fluorosis, but the majority of cases are mild and do not cause serious effects.

Extremely high doses of fluoride can cause vomiting, diarrhea, and even death, but it would be nearly impossible to get toxic amounts from water or dental products. The UL for fluoride is currently set at 10 mg for individuals nine years and older.

DID YOU KNOW?

As of 2016, more than 62% of Americans get their tap water from fluoridated municipal water systems.

MINERAL TIPS

Fluoride is not usually added to bottled water, neither is there a requirement for it to appear on the label. The FDA is currently working on establishing a limit of 0.7 mg per liter for fluoride added to bottled water.

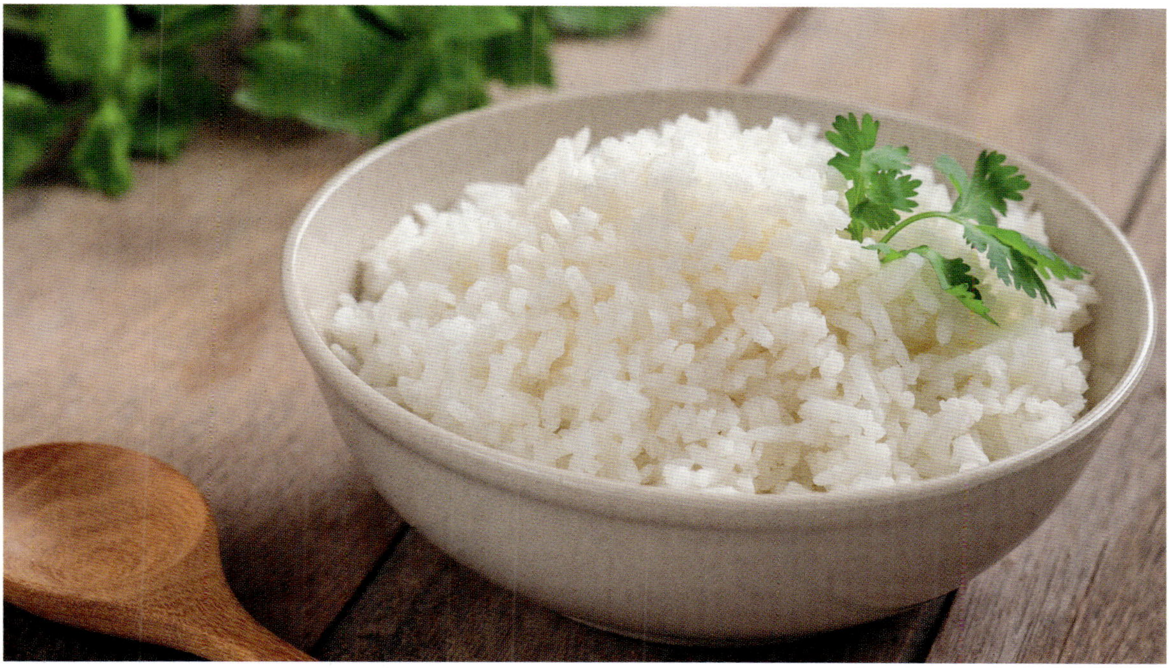

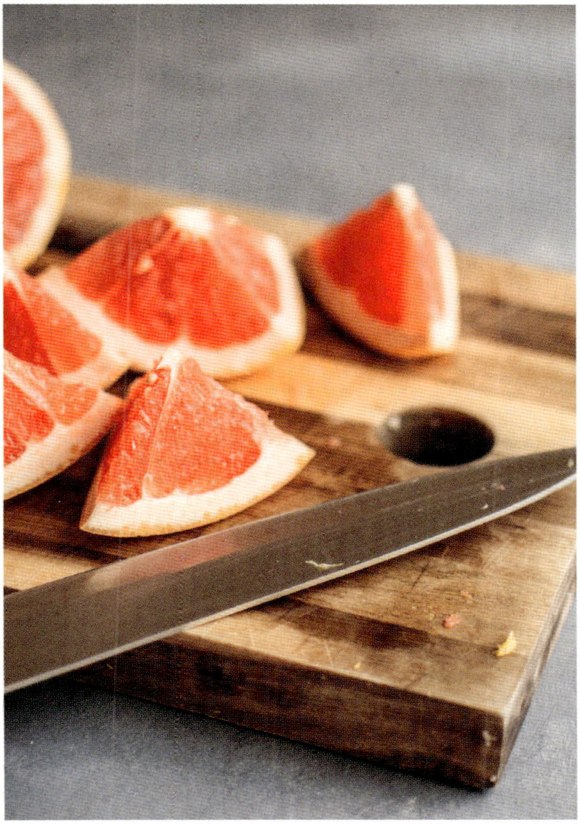

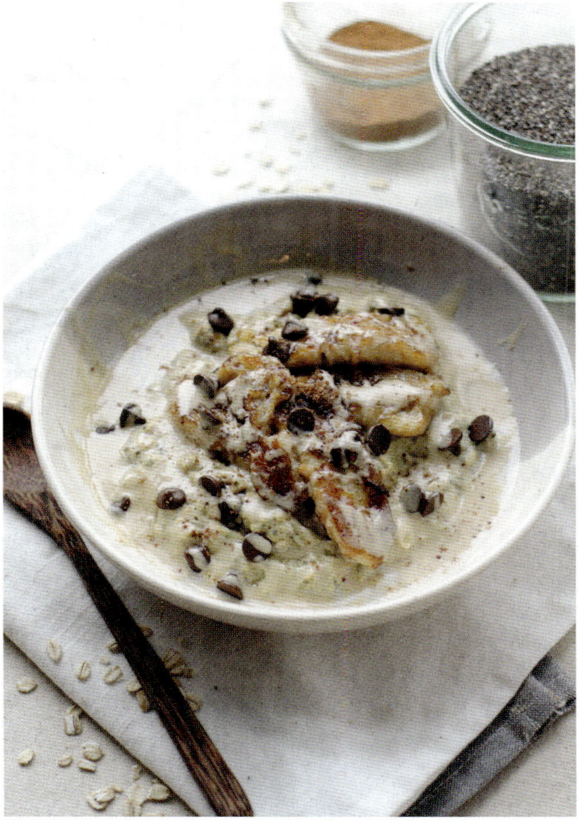

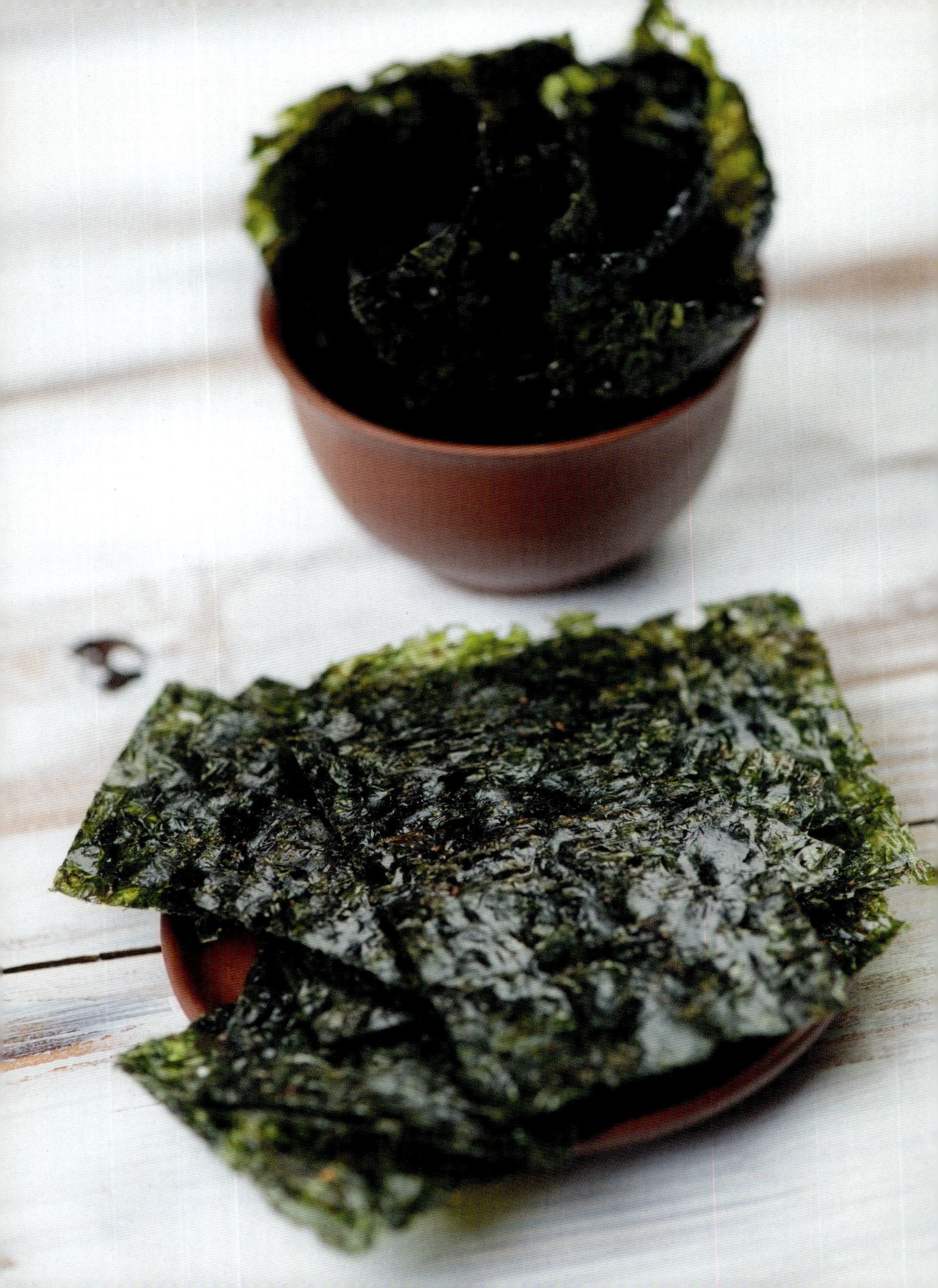

[IODINE]

THE **THYROID** HELPER

RECOMMENDED DIETARY ALLOWANCE (RDA)

Men and women	150 mcg
Pregnancy	220 mcg
Lactation	290 mcg

Did you know that Appalachian regions and areas surrounding the Great Lakes in the Midwest were once known as the "goiter belt"?

AIDING THYROID FUNCTION

This nickname stemmed from the high prevalence of iodine deficiency in people living in these areas, mostly due to the erosion of iodine in the soil used to grow foods. A characteristic sign of deficiency is the enlargement of the thyroid gland at the base of the neck, known as a goiter.

As with most nutrients, what happens as a result of inadequate intake provides a glimpse into the important functions of iodine in the body. This essential mineral is part of thyroid hormones that regulate growth, brain development, metabolism, and reproduction. While iodine deficiency is no longer an issue in the United States, thanks to the iodization of salt in the 1920s, more than 30% of the world's population may be at risk of deficiency.

COMMON FOOD SOURCES

Iodine is present in seawater, so seafood and seaweed are good sources of this mineral. It's also found in eggs, dairy, and some plant foods. The iodine content of foods largely depends on the level of this nutrient in soils used to grow crops. Just three ounces of baked cod provides enough iodine to meet daily needs.

Nori seaweed (10 g, dried)	232 mcg*
Cod (3 oz, baked)	158 mcg
Greek yogurt (1 cup, nonfat)	116 mcg
Oysters (3 oz, cooked)	93 mcg
Iodized table salt (about 1/4 tsp)	76 mcg
Potato (1 medium, baked)	60 mcg
Navy beans (1/2 cup, cooked)	32 mcg
Egg (1 large, hard-boiled)	26 mcg
Chocolate ice cream (1/2 cup)	21 mcg
Shrimp (3 oz, cooked)	13 mcg

* Could be as high as 2,984 mcg/g

ROLE IN THE BODY

Since iodine is an important component of T3 and T4 thyroid hormones, it's necessary for normal thyroid function. The thyroid controls body temperature, metabolism, growth, and reproduction. During iodine deficiency, the enlargement of the thyroid gland into a goiter occurs as the body tries to maximize the uptake of iodine in the body. Severe deficiency can result in hypothyroidism, marked by fatigue, increased sensitivity to cold, hair loss, weight gain, and more.

Iodine also plays a vital role in the proper neurodevelopment of children. Iodine deficiency during pregnancy can cause intellectual disabilities, stunted growth, and delays in sexual maturation.

USING SUPPLEMENTS

Iodine exists on its own in supplements and in many multivitamin/minerals and prenatal vitamins. Taking iodine supplements is unnecessary if you have adequate dietary intake. Excess iodine can also cause the development of a goiter and may lead to iodine-induced hyperthyroidism. The UL for iodine is 1,100 mcg, but it's unlikely for anyone to get this much iodine from food or supplements, with the exception of some seaweed snacks.

NOTES ON DEFICIENCY

Dietary iodine intake is considered adequate in the United States, but there are still some groups at risk of insufficiency. People who do not use iodized salt, vegans, and those living in areas with iodine-deficient soils may have a higher chance of developing iodine deficiency. Using iodized salt and increasing intake of iodine-rich foods is the best way to prevent deficiency.

DID YOU KNOW?

Highly processed and canned foods tend to have salt added, so you may think they're high in iodine. However, this salt is almost always non-iodized.

MINERAL TIPS

Most table salt in the United States is iodized, but sea salt, Kosher salt, fleur de sel, and pink Himalayan salt, do not typically contain added iodine. Even though it comes from seawater, non-iodized sea salt has essentially no naturally occurring iodine.

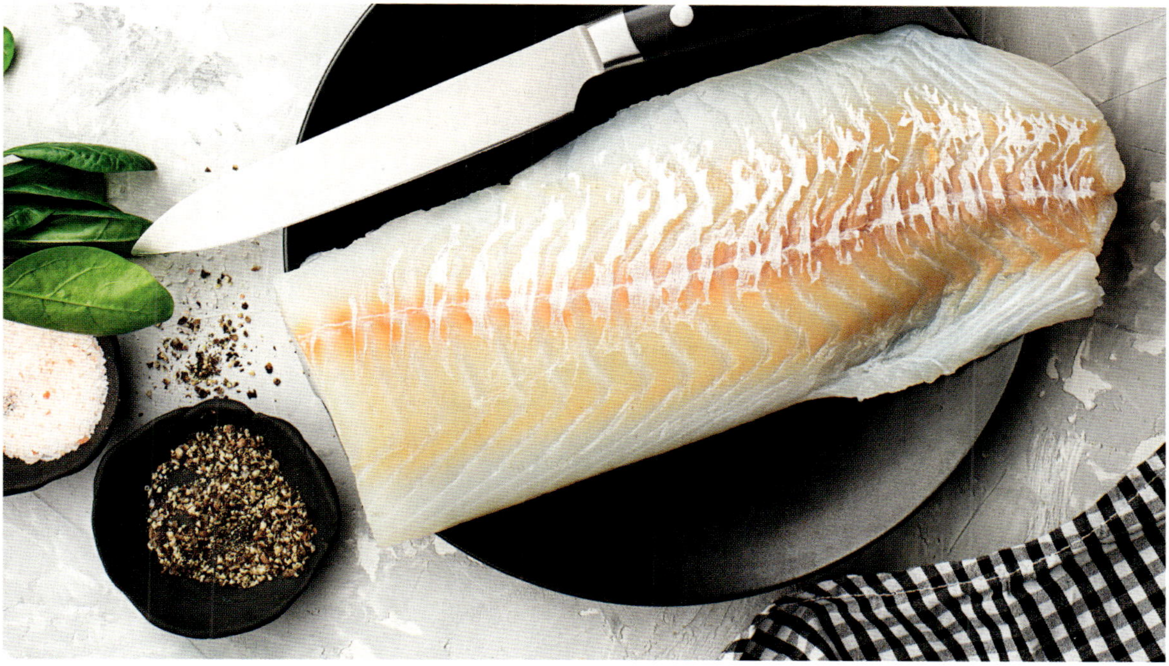

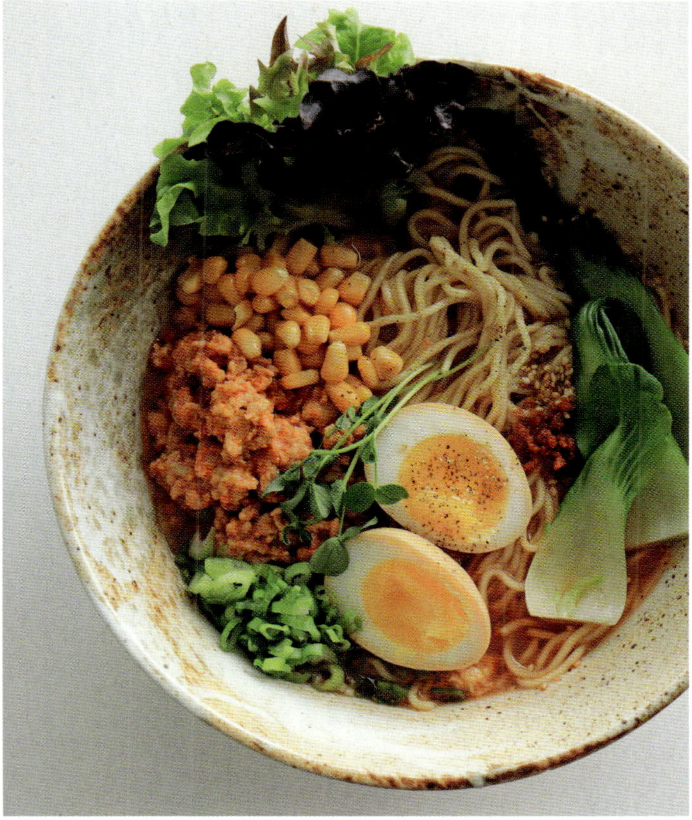

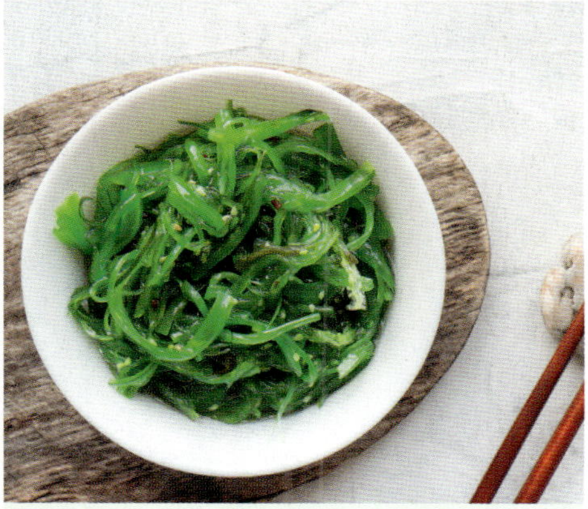

IN THE KITCHEN

SEAWEED SALAD

Soak a $^{3}/_{4}$-oz sheet of dried seaweed in warm water for a few minutes. Whisk together $^{1}/_{4}$ cup each of rice vinegar and soy sauce, 1 tbsp toasted sesame oil, 1 tsp chopped ginger, and a pinch of red pepper flakes. Drain the seaweed, slice into smaller pieces if needed, and toss in the dressing.

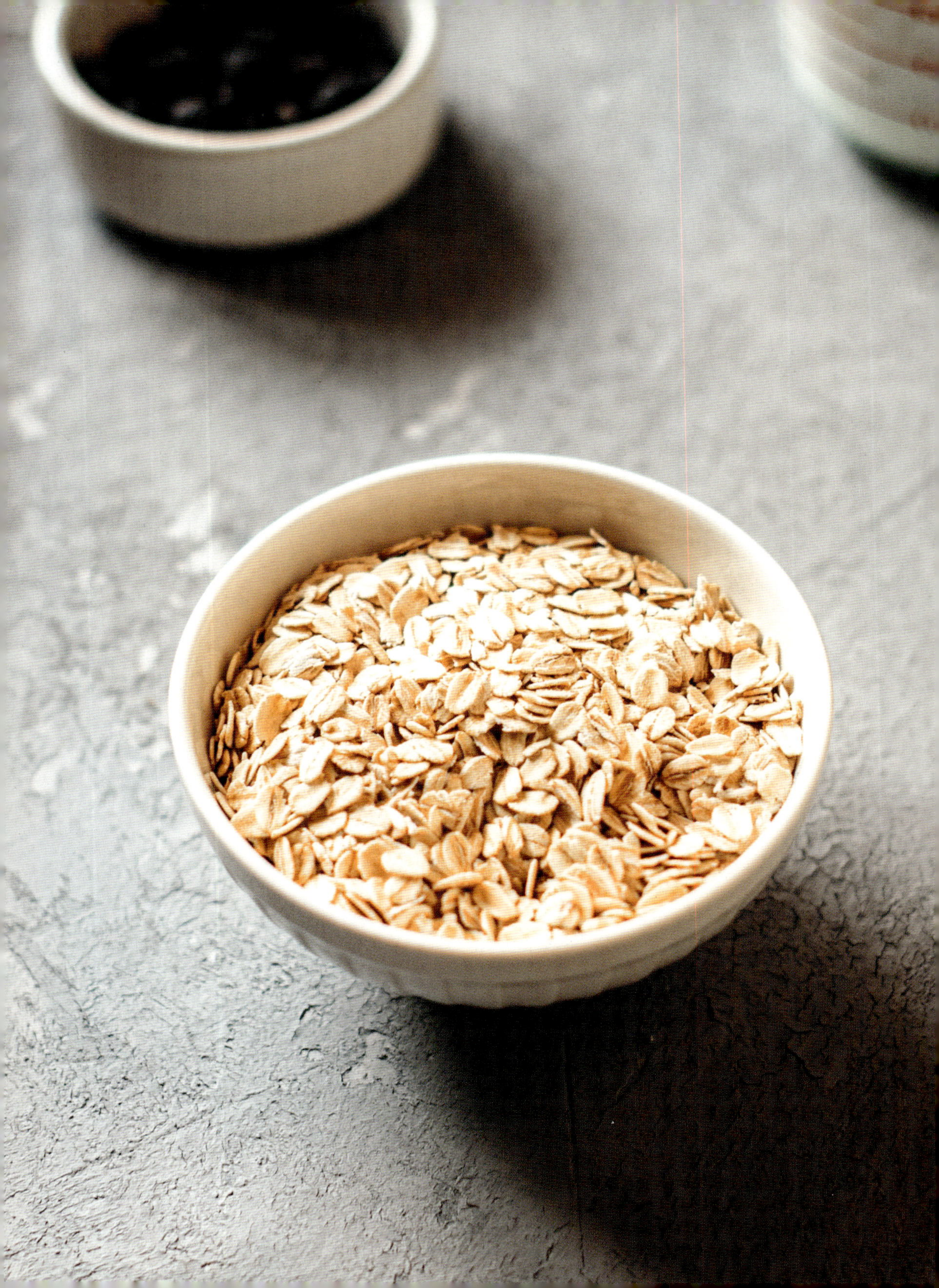

[IRON]

THE **BLOOD** BUILDER

RECOMMENDED DIETARY ALLOWANCE (RDA)

Men (19–50 years)	8 mg
Women (19–50 years)	18 mg
Men and women (51+ years)	8 mg
Pregnancy	27 mg
Lactation (14–18 years)	10 mg
Lactation (19–50 years)	9 mg

Many people may think of spinach as a rich source of iron, thanks to the cartoon character Popeye, but it's not as good a source as you may think. In 1870, a scientist made a decimal error when reporting the iron content of spinach, suggesting that 100 grams had 35 mg instead of the actual 3.5 mg.

Iron is needed in smaller amounts than some other minerals, but has important functions in the body. Adequate intake is essential for proper growth, brain development, and the transfer of oxygen in the blood. Women need more iron during pregnancy and lactation to support infant growth. Women also have higher needs during their reproductive years, in part to account for iron lost through menstrual bleeding.

HEME AND NONHEME IRON

In foods, iron exists in two forms: heme and nonheme. Meats and seafood contain both heme and nonheme forms, while plant foods and iron-fortified products only have nonheme iron. Heme iron is more readily absorbed than nonheme forms, in part because nonheme iron absorption is affected by other nutrients present in the same meal.

COMMON FOOD SOURCES

A bowl of iron-fortified oatmeal provides enough iron for women to meet their daily needs, while a cup of lentils and a handful of cashews has a day's worth of iron for men.

Oatmeal (1/2 cup, fortified, dry)	20 mg
Spinach (1 cup, boiled)	6.4 mg
Lentils (1 cup, cooked)	6 mg
Ground beef (1 cup, cooked)	3 mg
Tofu (1/2 cup, firm)	3 mg
Tomatoes (1/2 cup, stewed)	2 mg
Sardines (3 oz, canned in oil, drained)	2 mg
Cashew nuts (1 oz, raw)	2 mg
Turkey breast (3 oz, roasted)	1 mg
Brown rice (1 cup, cooked)	1 mg
Pecans (1 oz, raw)	0.7 mg

ROLE IN THE BODY

Iron is a component of both hemoglobin and myoglobin. Hemoglobin is a protein that delivers oxygen from the lungs to tissues in the body; the protein myoglobin carries oxygen in muscle tissue.

Certain enzymes that play an important role in the creation of ATP, a compound that carries energy in cells, also contain iron. Thus, this mineral is vital to the metabolism and production of energy.

Adequate iron status is also necessary for healthy pregnancies and proper growth throughout the life cycle. Infants and young children who do not receive enough iron may be at risk of impaired growth as well as intellectual and motor development.

USING SUPPLEMENTS

Iron supplements are helpful for some people, including pregnant women and individuals with inadequate intake, but you shouldn't take them unless it's necessary. Too much supplemental iron can cause nausea, constipation, and possibly even organ damage. The UL is 45 mg per day.

NOTES ON DEFICIENCY

Supplements are often recommended to prevent and correct deficiency in vulnerable populations. There are also ways to boost iron absorption through diet. For example, vitamin C, heme iron from animal foods, and beta-carotene enhance the absorption of nonheme iron.

Who's at risk?

Populations at risk of iron-deficiency anemia include menstruating and pregnant women, children, frequent blood donors, and individuals following a predominantly plant-based diet.

What are the symptoms

Symptoms of anemia include fatigue, shortness of breath, fast heartbeat, lightheadedness, increased sensitivity to cold, and pale skin.

Caution for vegans and vegetarians

The RDA for iron is 1.8 times higher for vegans and vegetarians. This is mostly because nonheme iron is not as well absorbed as heme iron. Plus, some plant foods may contain compounds that bind to iron and make it harder to absorb. Phytates, present in grains and beans, and polyphenols, found in varying degrees in fruits, vegetables, tea, coffee, and wine, inhibit iron absorption.

DID YOU KNOW?

Iron deficiency is the most common nutrient deficiency in the world. The body is better at absorbing iron when you are deficient than when you have adequate stores.

MINERAL TIPS

Boost iron intake from plant foods by eating them with a source of vitamin C, such as citrus, bell peppers, and strawberries.

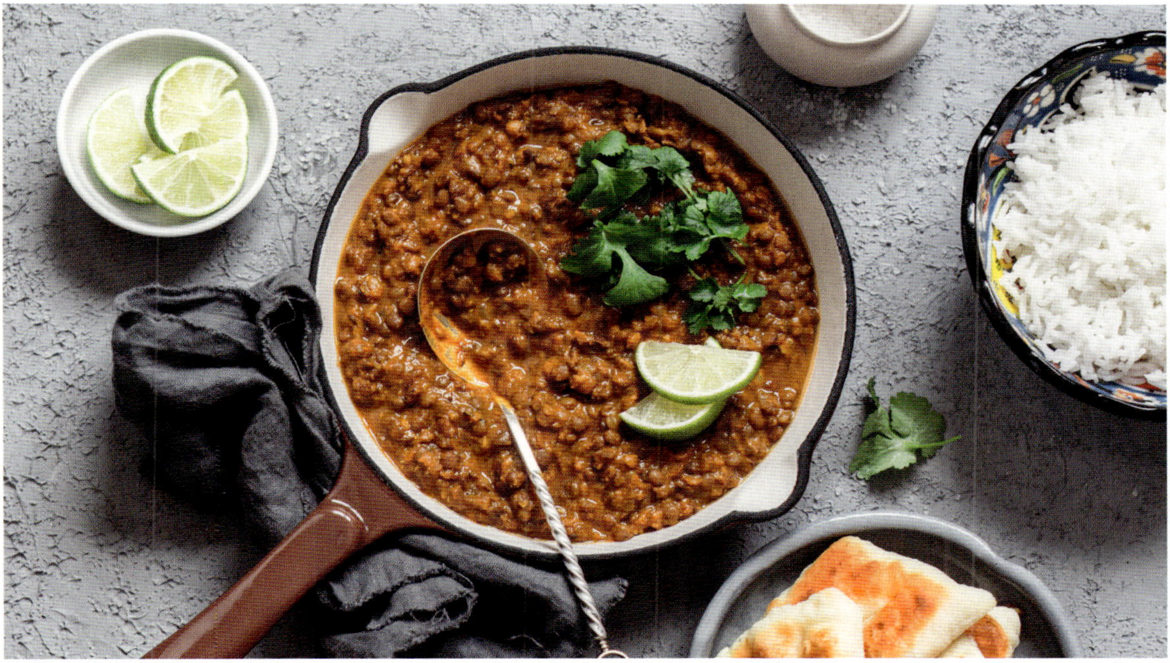

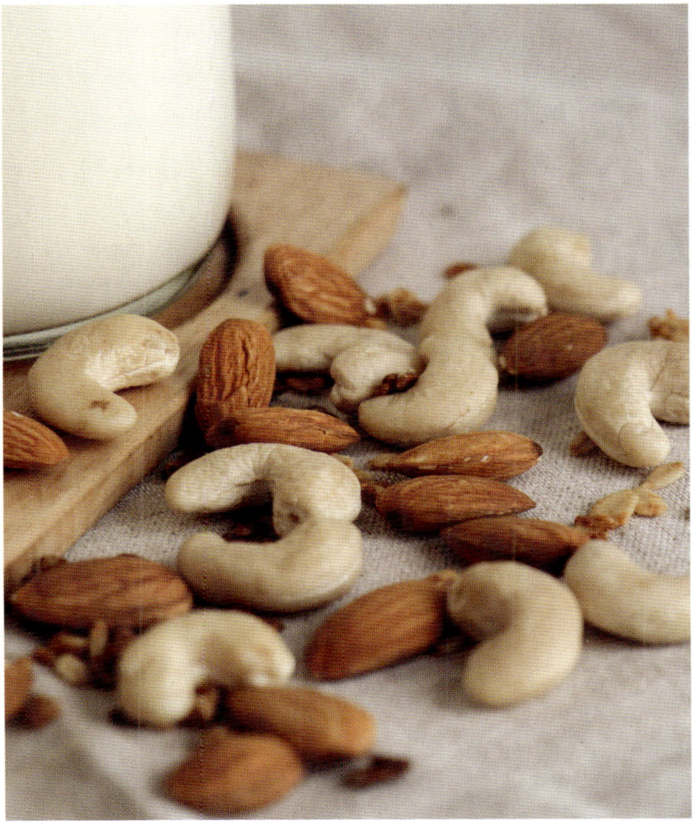

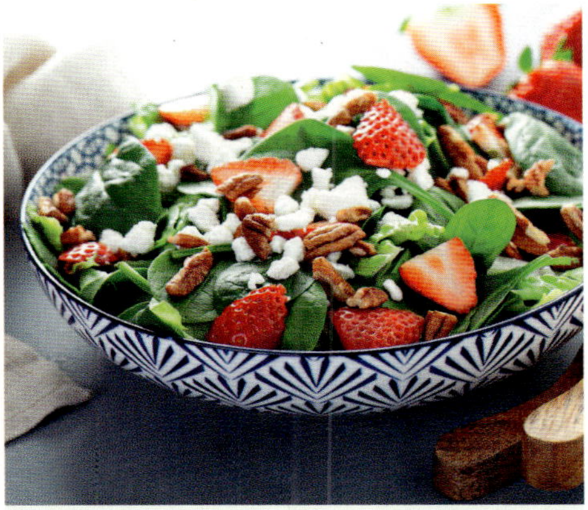

IN THE KITCHEN
SALAD BOWL

Try a spinach salad with strawberries, goat cheese, pecans, and lemon vinaigrette for an iron-rich dish.

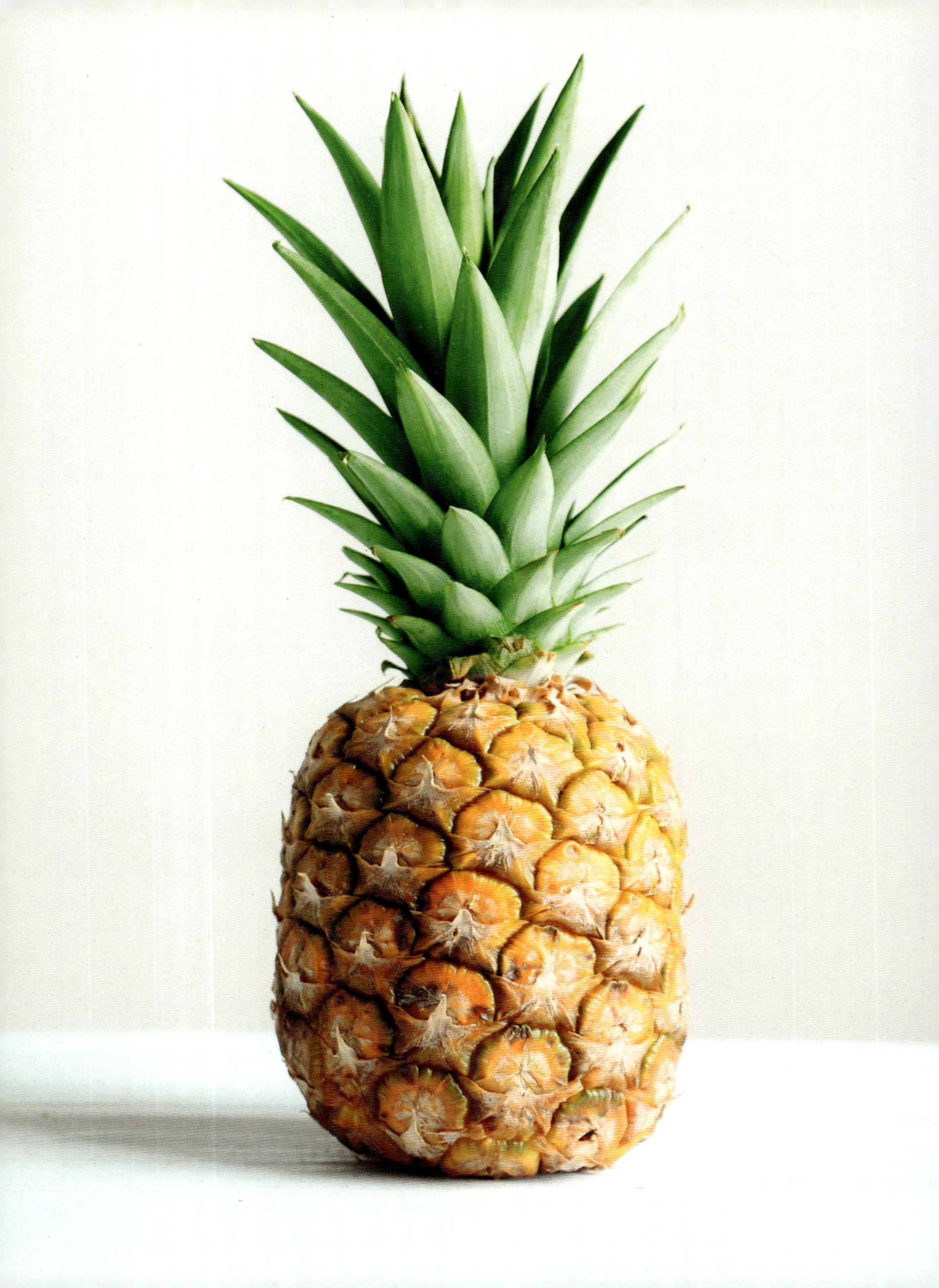

[MANGANESE]

THE **MITOCHONDRIA** PROTECTOR

ADEQUATE INTAKE (AI)

Men	2.3 mg
Women	1.8 mg
Pregnancy	2 mg
Lactation	2.6 mg

Let's take a moment to step back in time to your middle school biology class. Does the term mitochondria—"powerhouse of the cell"—ring a bell? You may remember that mitochondria are responsible for turning energy from food into energy that cells can use, but you probably don't know that manganese is very important for supporting mitochondrial health.

Manganese is a trace mineral that's essential for human health. Some of the functions of manganese and symptoms of deficiency are not fully understood. However, it's thought that this nutrient plays an important role in bone development and wound healing.

COMMON FOOD SOURCES

Meeting daily manganese needs is easy to do if you eat a predominantly plant-based diet. Some of the richest sources of manganese include whole grains, leafy vegetables, some fruits, and nuts. Two cups of pineapple provide more than enough manganese for one day.

Hazelnuts (1 oz, roasted)	1.6 mg
Pecans (1 oz, roasted)	1.1 mg
Brown rice (1/2 cup, cooked)	1.07 mg
Clams (3 oz, cooked)	0.9 mg
Pineapple (1/2 cup, chunks)	0.8 mg
Soybeans (1/2 cup, boiled)	0.7 mg
Black tea (1 cup)	0.5 mg
Pinto beans (1/2 cup, cooked)	0.39 mg
Acorn squash (1/2 cup, cooked)	0.3 mg

ROLE IN THE BODY

As an essential component of the antioxidant enzyme manganese superoxide dismutase (MnSOD), manganese is vital to protecting mitochondria from oxidative stress. It's also a cofactor for enzymes that facilitate bone and cartilage formation, as well as the enzyme that helps provide the building blocks of collagen for human skin.

Limited research suggests that decreased levels of manganese may increase the risk of developing osteoporosis or diabetes. However, the results of studies have been mixed, and there's no strong evidence that correcting low levels of manganese with supplements is beneficial.

USING SUPPLEMENTS

There's no need for manganese supplements if you eat a varied diet. Manganese toxicity can cause irreversible damage to the central nervous system, as well as mania, depression, irritability, and neurological symptoms similar to Parkinson's disease. However, toxicity has not been reported from dietary intake. It has only occurred in individuals exposed to high amounts of manganese dust in the workplace and manganese-contaminated drinking water. The UL for manganese is 11 mg per day.

DID YOU KNOW?

Magnesium and manganese are both named after the Magnesia region of Greece, where the two minerals were first isolated.

NOTES ON DEFICIENCY

Manganese deficiency is rare. Not much is known about the signs and symptoms of deficiency, but limited reports suggest that it could lead to bone demineralization, skin rashes, and low blood cholesterol.

MINERAL TIPS

Tannins in tea and phytic acid in beans, seeds, nuts, soybeans, and whole grains may slightly reduce manganese absorption. If you eat a balanced diet with a variety of foods that contain manganese, this should not be a major concern.

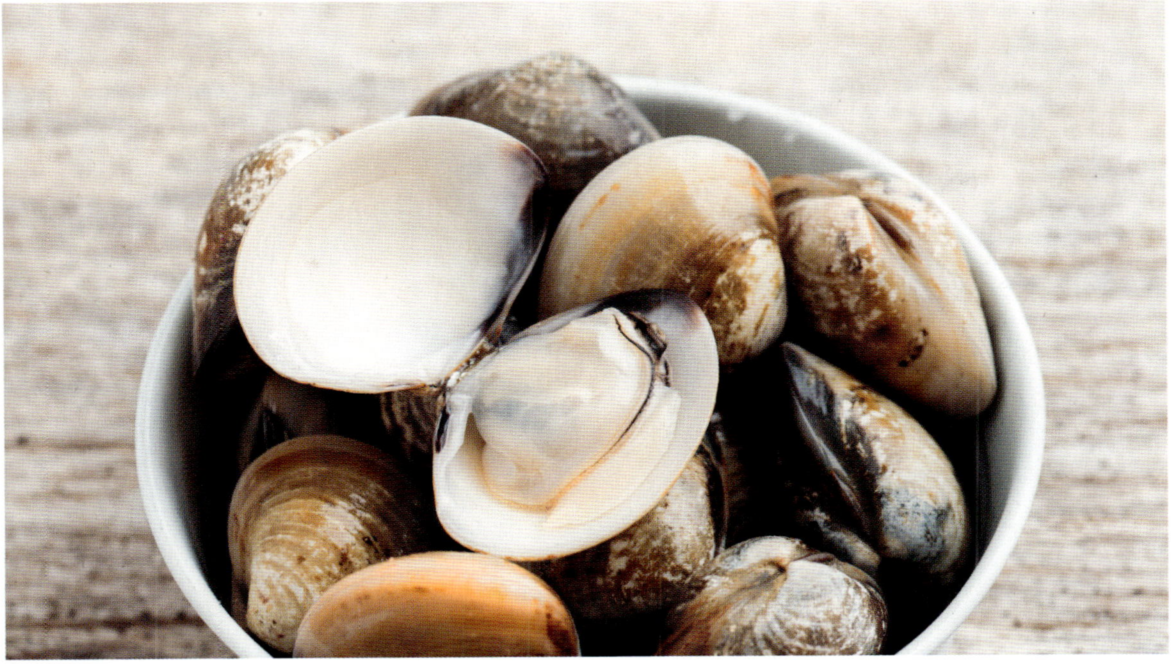

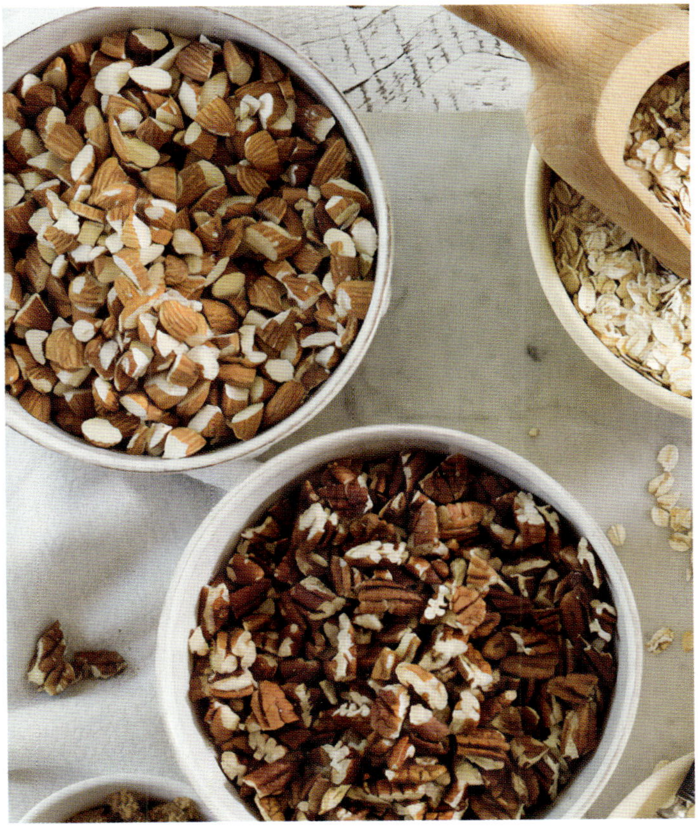

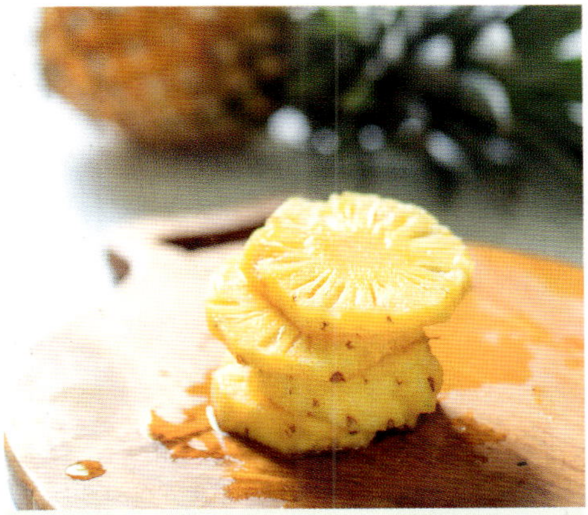

IN THE KITCHEN

PINEAPPLE FRIED RICE

In a skillet, sauté 1 cup chopped pineapple, 1 handful chopped green onions, 1 diced bell pepper, and some minced garlic in 2 tbsp olive oil. Add 1/2 cup brown rice and cook for a few minutes until warmed through. Serve with a protein of your choice—beans, scrambled eggs, or shredded chicken.

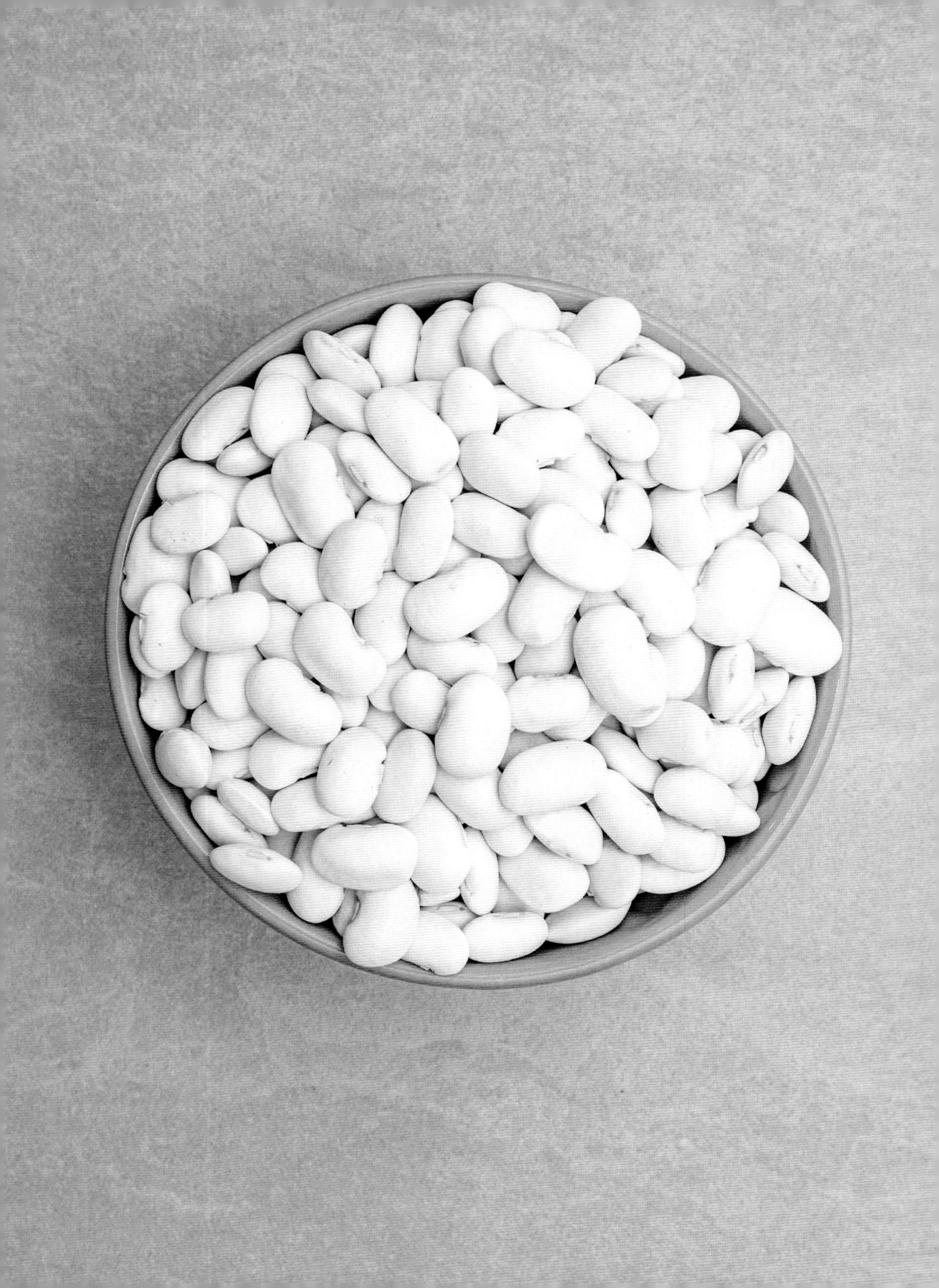

[MOLYBDENUM]

THE **"DIRTY"** NUTRIENT

RECOMMENDED DIETARY ALLOWANCE (RDA)

Men and women	45 mcg
Pregnancy and lactation	50 mcg

Many people may not realize how strongly the composition of soil dictates the nutritional profile of some foods. This is especially the case for molybdenum, an essential trace mineral that enters various foods via the dirt and water used in agriculture.

SOIL COMPOSITION

Not surprisingly, the molybdenum content of foods varies widely depending on location. But even with variations in soil composition, molybdenum is present in a wide variety of foods. Whereas some regions were particularly prone to iodine deficiency due to nutrient-poor soil before the iodization of salt, the typical American diet provides more than enough molybdenum.

COMMON FOOD SOURCES

The best food sources of molybdenum include legumes, whole grains, and nuts. Fruits and vegetables generally have smaller amounts of this mineral. Just half a cup of black-eyed peas contains almost a week's worth of molybdenum.

Black-eyed peas (1/2 cup, boiled)	288 mcg
Lima beans (1/2 cup, boiled)	104 mcg
Plain yogurt (1 cup, low-fat)	26 mcg
Cheerios cereal (1/2 cup)	15 mcg
Banana (1 medium)	15 mcg
Whole wheat bread (1 slice)	12 mcg
Ground beef (3 oz, pan-fried)	8 mcg
Sweet corn (1/2 cup, cooked)	6 mcg

ROLE IN THE BODY

Molybdenum is a component of four enzymes that have functions ranging from the metabolism of sulfur amino acids to the processing of drugs and toxins. It also assists in the breakdown of the building blocks of DNA and RNA, which increase antioxidants in the blood.

As part of a compound known as tetrathiomolybdate (TM), molybdenum also plays a role in regulating copper status. TM binds to copper and prevents its absorption. Therefore, TM therapies are administered to individuals with Wilson's disease that have copper accumulation in tissues that leads to brain and liver damage.

Pilot studies also suggest that TM therapy may help prevent cancer progression. This concept is still being investigated, and the exact mechanism by which TM works is unclear. It's thought that by binding to copper, TM inhibits inflammation reactions that may increase cancer progression and rely on copper-dependent enzymes.

USING SUPPLEMENTS

You don't need to worry about taking molybdenum supplements if you eat a varied diet, and deficiency is not a concern for healthy adults. The UL for molybdenum is very high compared to the RDA—2,000 mcg for adults.

DID YOU KNOW?

After molybdenum was recognized as essential for human health in 1953, it took 18 years for more functions of this mineral to be identified.

NOTES ON DEFICIENCY

There are no reports of deficiency in healthy individuals.

MINERAL TIPS

The body can get rid of molybdenum quickly in the urine, so a high dietary intake of molybdenum poses no concerns.

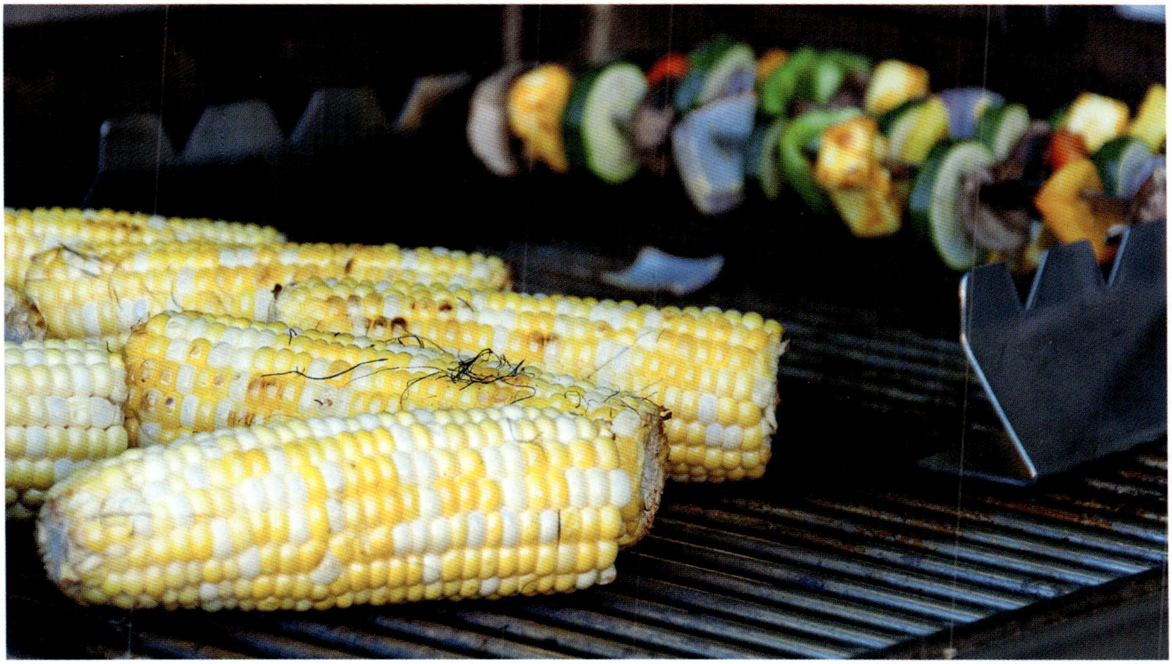

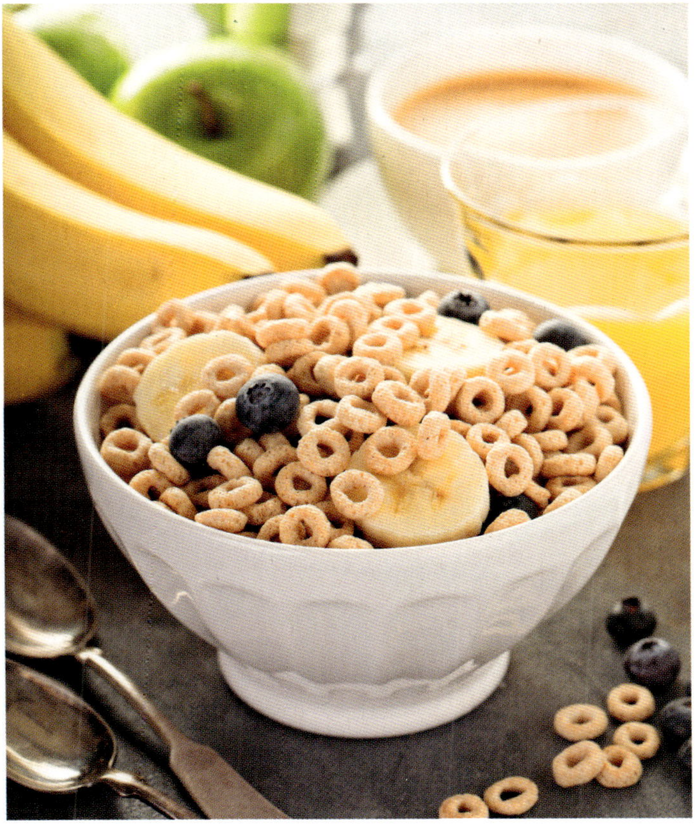

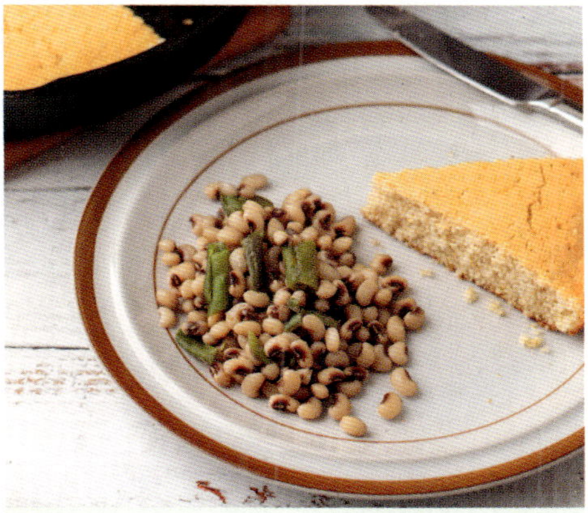

IN THE KITCHEN

A BOWL OF BLACK-EYED PEAS

Soak 1 lb dried black-eyed peas in water for at least 6 hours. Drain and rinse the black-eyed peas, and add them to a large pot with 6 cups chicken or vegetable stock. Bring to a boil, cover, and simmer for 45 minutes until tender. Stir in cooked chopped green beans before serving.

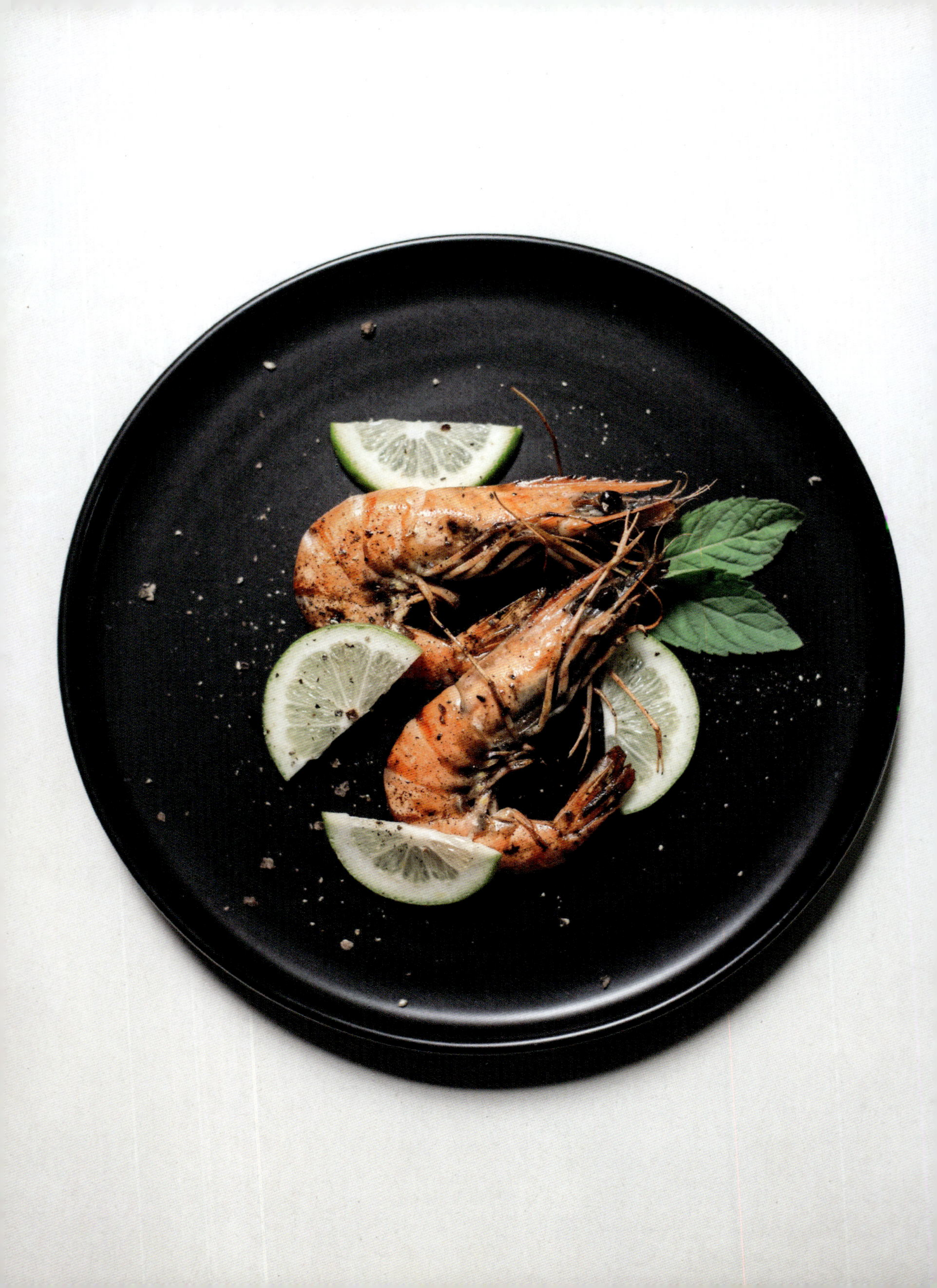

[SELENIUM]

THE **ANTIOXIDANT** MINERAL

RECOMMENDED DIETARY ALLOWANCE (RDA)

Men and women	55 mcg
Pregnancy	60 mcg
Lactation	70 mcg

Even though it's needed in small amounts, don't be fooled into thinking that selenium doesn't have many important roles.

ANTIOXIDANT MINERAL

This mineral is vital to the body's antioxidant functions, and selenium status may influence the risk of developing some chronic diseases.

Similar to other essential trace minerals, the selenium content of soil largely dictates how much of this nutrient is found in plant-based foods. But with so many selenium-rich food choices, it's not difficult to meet your daily needs. Interestingly, selenium makes its way into plants that have sulfur compounds, so garlic and Brassica vegetables such as broccoli and cabbage accumulate more selenium than other plants.

COMMON FOOD SOURCES

Grains, nuts, seeds, seafood, and meats provide selenium. A single Brazil nut contains more than enough of the RDA for selenium, but keep in mind that a serving of these nuts (about an ounce) has more than the UL.

Brazil nuts (1 oz/about 6 nuts)	544 mcg
Halibut (3 oz, cooked)	47 mcg
Shrimp (3 oz, grilled)	42 mcg
Ham (3 oz, roasted)	42 mcg
Macaroni (1 cup, enriched, cooked)	37 mcg
Turkey (3 oz, roasted)	31 mcg
1% cottage cheese (1 cup)	20 mcg
Sunflower seeds (1/4 cup, dried)	19 mcg
Marinara sauce (1 cup)	4 mcg
Lentils (1 cup, boiled)	6 mcg

ROLE IN THE BODY

Selenium is part of at least 25 selenoproteins, several of which are known to play key roles in the creation of thyroid hormone, DNA synthesis, and antioxidant functions.

One category of these proteins, known as glutathione peroxidases, helps reduce reactive oxygen species that can damage cells and are vital in male fertility and sperm production. Other selenium-containing proteins regulate thyroid function by converting thyroid hormone into its active form. The thyroid controls metabolism and body temperature regulation.

The importance of selenium in the body may suggest that it can help prevent disease development. Observational studies have found an inverse association between blood selenium levels and the risk of high blood pressure. Selenium status may also impact immunity, and deficiency in the mineral has been linked to chronic inflammation and weakened immune response.

USING SUPPLEMENTS

There are many types of selenium supplements on the market, but they're not usually recommended for the average adult. Selenium toxicity can cause significant side effects, including brittle hair and nails, skin rashes, garlic breath, and neurological disorders. The UL for selenium from food and supplements is 400 mcg per day.

NOTES ON DEFICIENCY

Overt selenium deficiency is rare in the United States, and most Americans get enough of this essential trace mineral from their diets. Prolonged inadequate selenium intake, even if deficiency is not obvious, may increase the body's susceptibility to stress.

DID YOU KNOW?

Risk of selenium deficiency is high in areas where selenium levels in soil are low and most of the population follows a vegetarian diet, such as in parts of China.

MINERAL TIPS

It's easy to meet your selenium needs, even if you don't eat Brazil nuts. Start your morning with a bowl of oatmeal sprinkled with sunflower seeds, and have some cottage cheese as a snack.

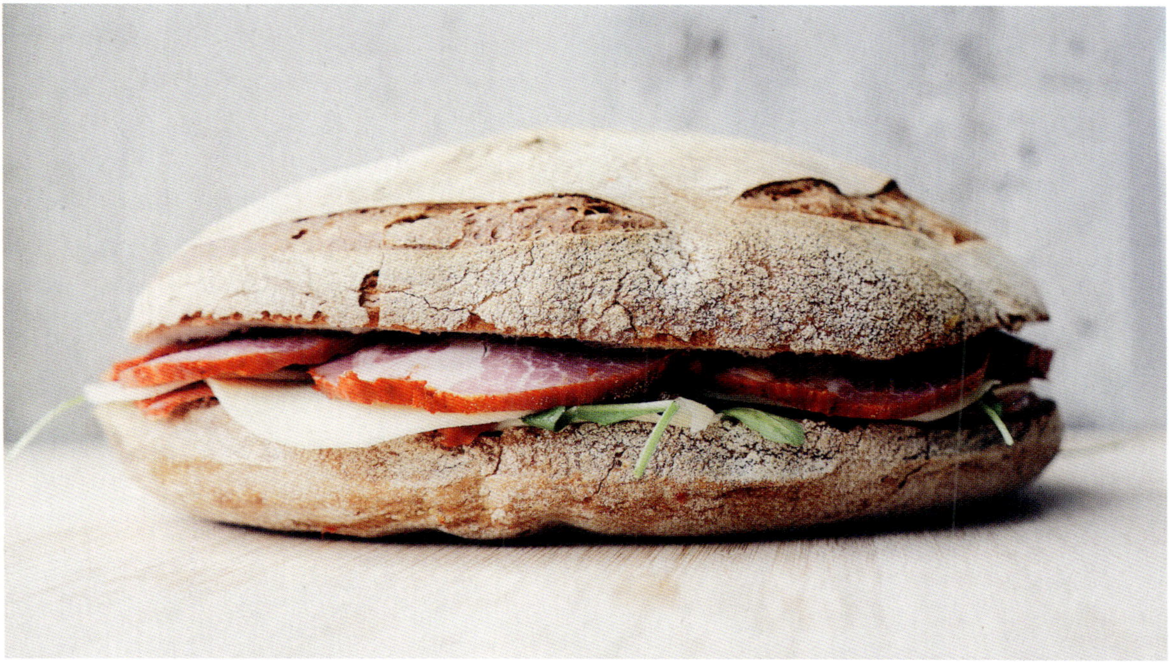

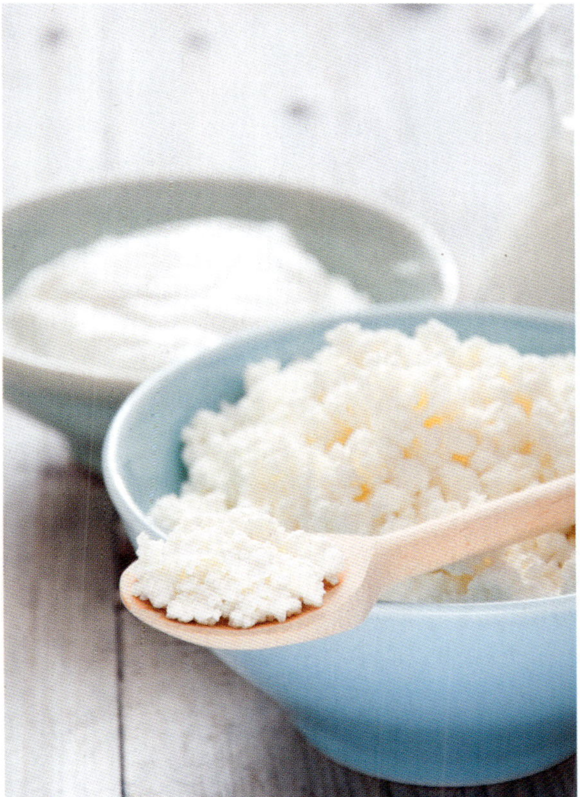

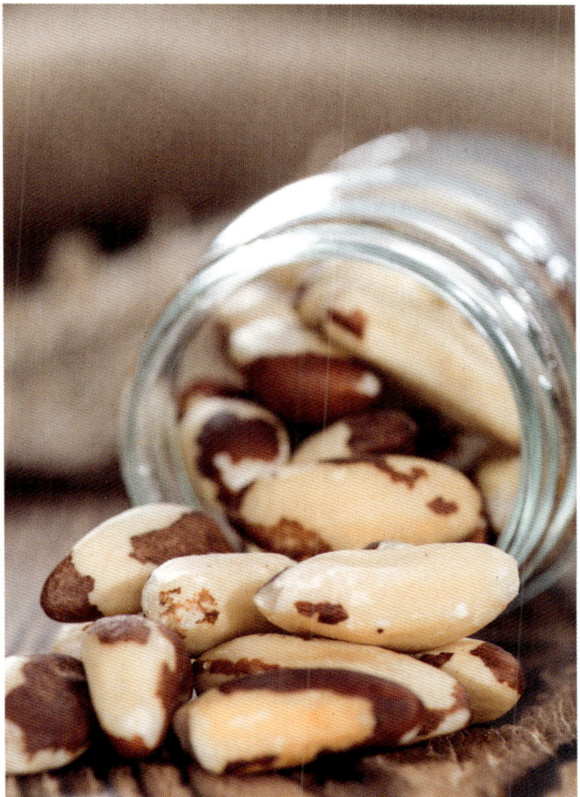

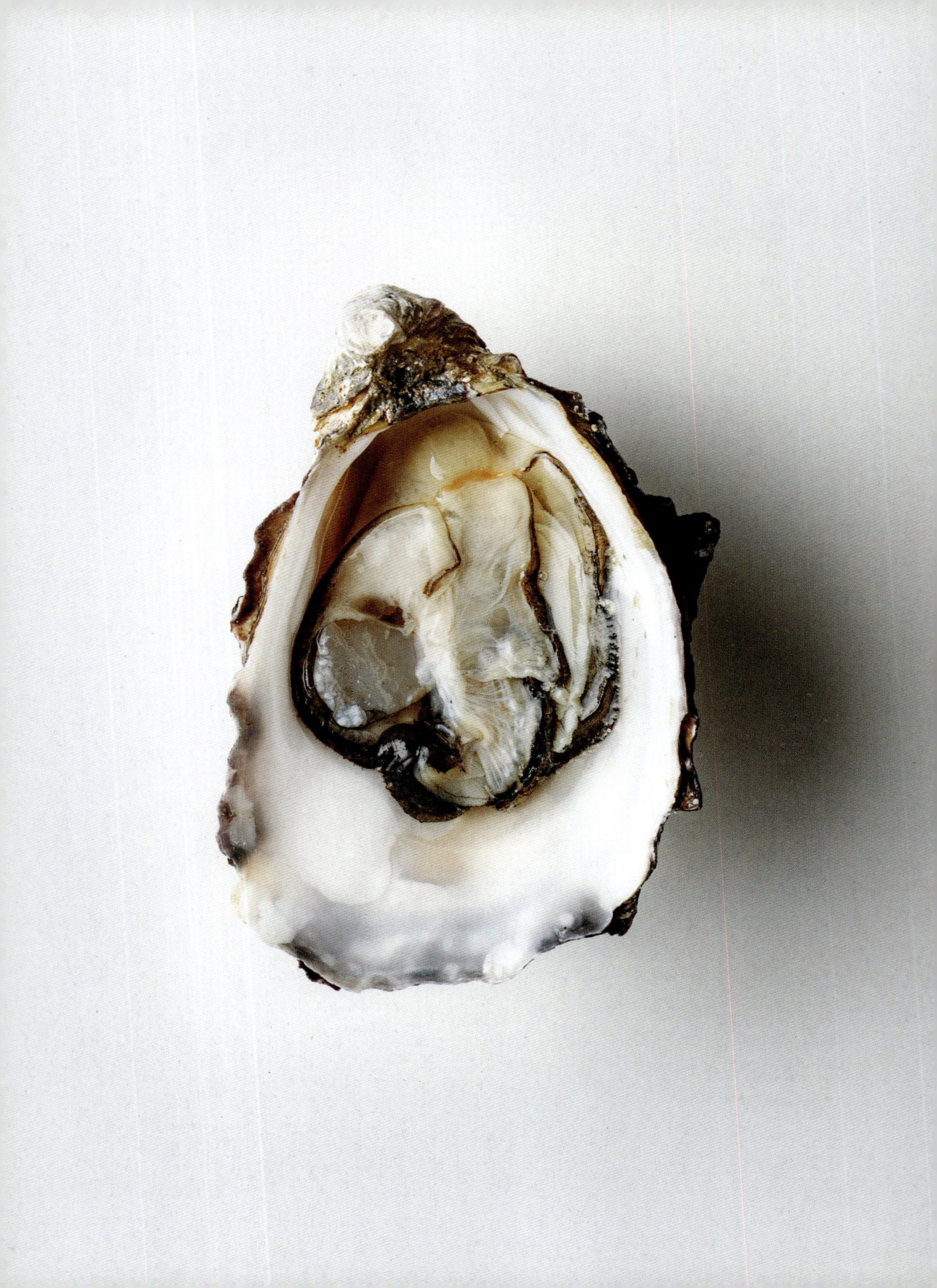

[ZINC]

THE **IMMUNITY** MINERAL

RECOMMENDED DIETARY ALLOWANCE (RDA)

Men	11 mg
Women	8 mg
Pregnancy (14-18 years)	12 mg
Lactation (14–18 years)	13 mg
Pregnancy (19+ years)	11 mg
Lactation (19+ years)	12 mg

If you consider the importance of nutrition at any stage in the life cycle, zinc takes a front seat in every phase.

A MINERAL FOR ALL AGES

This mineral is vital for healthy pregnancies, growth and development during childhood and adolescence, and immune system function throughout life but especially during older adulthood. It's also necessary for having a proper sense of smell and taste.

Most Americans get enough zinc from their diets, but developing countries have higher rates of zinc deficiency. The zinc in whole grains and other plant-based foods is not well absorbed, since phytates can bind to zinc and inhibit absorption. Fortunately, there are many other zinc-rich foods that you can eat to meet your needs.

COMMON FOOD SOURCES

Oysters, nuts, and beans are good sources of zinc. However, due to the presence of phytates in most plant-based sources of zinc, the body may not absorb zinc from plants as well as from animal products. Three ounces of oysters have close to 700% of daily zinc needs.

Oysters (3 oz, fried)	74 mg
Alaska king crab (3 oz, cooked)	6.5 mg
Lobster (3 oz, cooked)	3.4 mg
Baked beans (1/2 cup, canned)	2.9 mg
Chicken (3 oz dark meat, cooked)	2.4 mg
Pumpkin seeds (1 oz, dried)	2.2 mg
Pine nuts (1 oz, raw)	1.8 mg
Fruit yogurt (1 cup, low-fat)	1.7 mg
Chickpeas (1/2 cup, cooked)	1.3 mg
Swiss cheese (1 oz)	1.2 mg
Green peas (1/2 cup, cooked)	0.5 mg

ROLE IN THE BODY

Zinc assists more than 100 enzymes in catalyzing reactions, and more than 3,000 proteins in the body have zinc-binding sites. By maintaining skin strength, zinc helps with the wound-healing process. It plays a role in repairing membranes, lowering inflammation, fighting oxidative stress, and reducing scar formation.

Getting enough zinc during pregnancy is paramount to proper fetal development, and deficiency during this time has been linked to birth defects, growth delays, and increased infection risk. Infants, children, and adolescents continue to need adequate zinc supplies to support growth, development, and sexual maturation.

Zinc is also necessary for proper immune function, and low zinc levels may worsen declines in immunity associated with aging. Elderly individuals with low blood zinc concentrations are at a higher risk of pneumonia. However, there is no strong evidence supporting the use of zinc supplements to boost immunity in older adults.

NOTES ON DEFICIENCY

Characteristics of zinc deficiency include appetite loss, delayed growth, impaired immunity, and even hair loss, diarrhea, delayed sexual maturation, and skin lesions in serious cases. Though rare in North America, certain groups may be at risk of deficiency or inadequacy. These include vegetarians and vegans, pregnant and lactating women, and individuals with alcoholism.

DID YOU KNOW?

Zinc from meat and fish is more available to the body, in part because these sources do not contain phytates that limit zinc absorption.

USING SUPPLEMENTS

Zinc is available in several forms in supplements and homeopathic remedies. It's not necessary to regularly take zinc supplements if you eat a balanced diet. However, some research suggests that zinc lozenges may reduce the duration of common cold symptoms. Long-term use and high doses of zinc supplements may lead to copper deficiency. The UL for zinc is 40 mg per day.

MINERAL TIPS

Due to the limited bioavailability of zinc from plant-based foods, vegetarians and vegans need up to 50% more than the RDA for zinc. Soak beans, grains, and seeds in water overnight before cooking to improve zinc bioavailability. Leavened breads contain more bioavailable zinc than unleavened bread products.

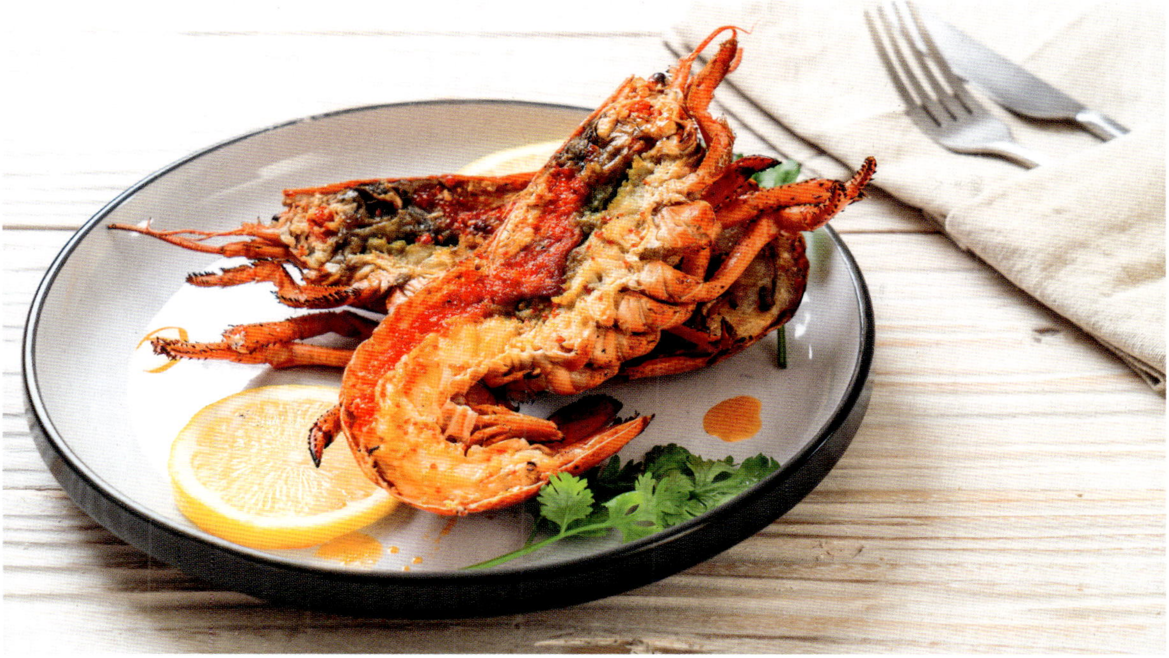

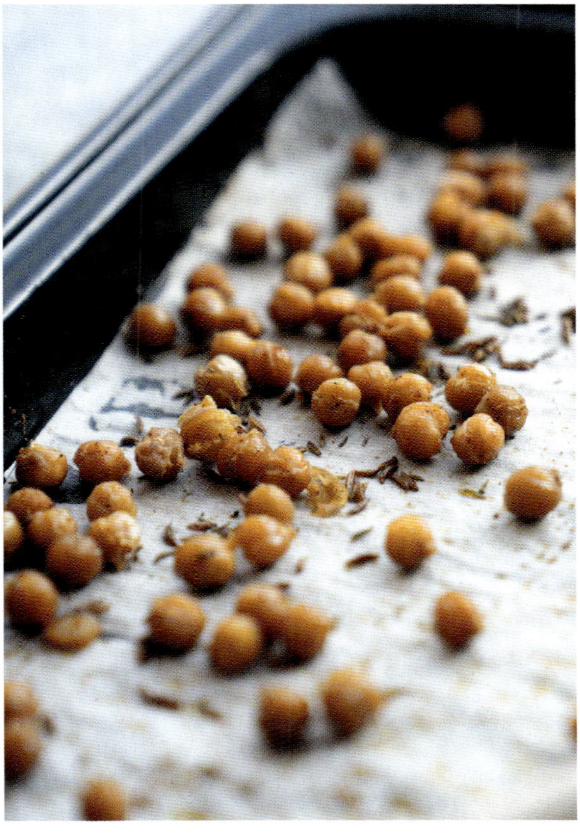

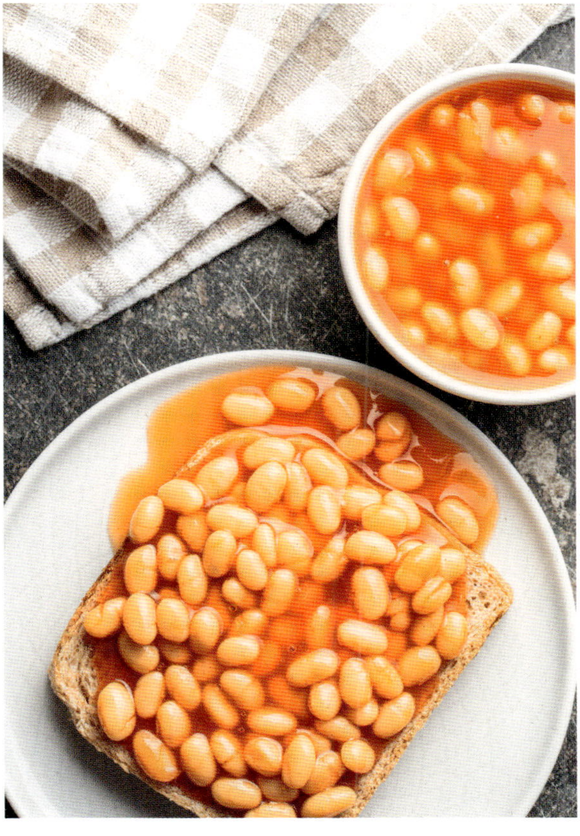

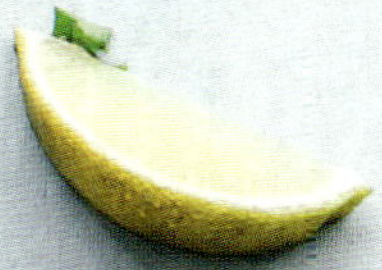

PART THREE: VITAMINS, MINERALS, AND YOU

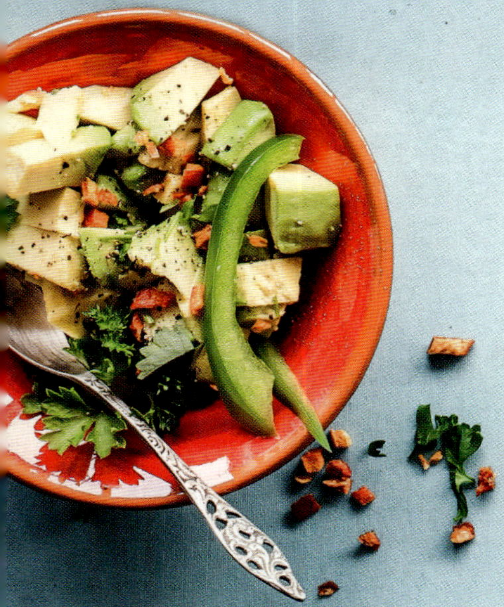

Now that you've learned about the essential micronutrients, it's time to discuss vitamins, minerals, and you. This section builds on the information in the previous chapters and includes common topics, questions, and concerns related to vitamins and minerals.

This section provides an insight into nutritional needs throughout the life cycle, nutrients of concern for health issues and special diets, and seasonal nutrition. You'll find lists of foods to eat by color, a review of the most nutrient-dense foods, and a sample weekly schedule to assist you in assessing the quality of your food choices. There's also a glossary of common supplements beyond vitamins and minerals and a feature on the hot topic of antioxidants. If you've ever wondered if vitamin D supplements live up to the hype or if it's really worth it to take multivitamins, the answers are on the upcoming pages.

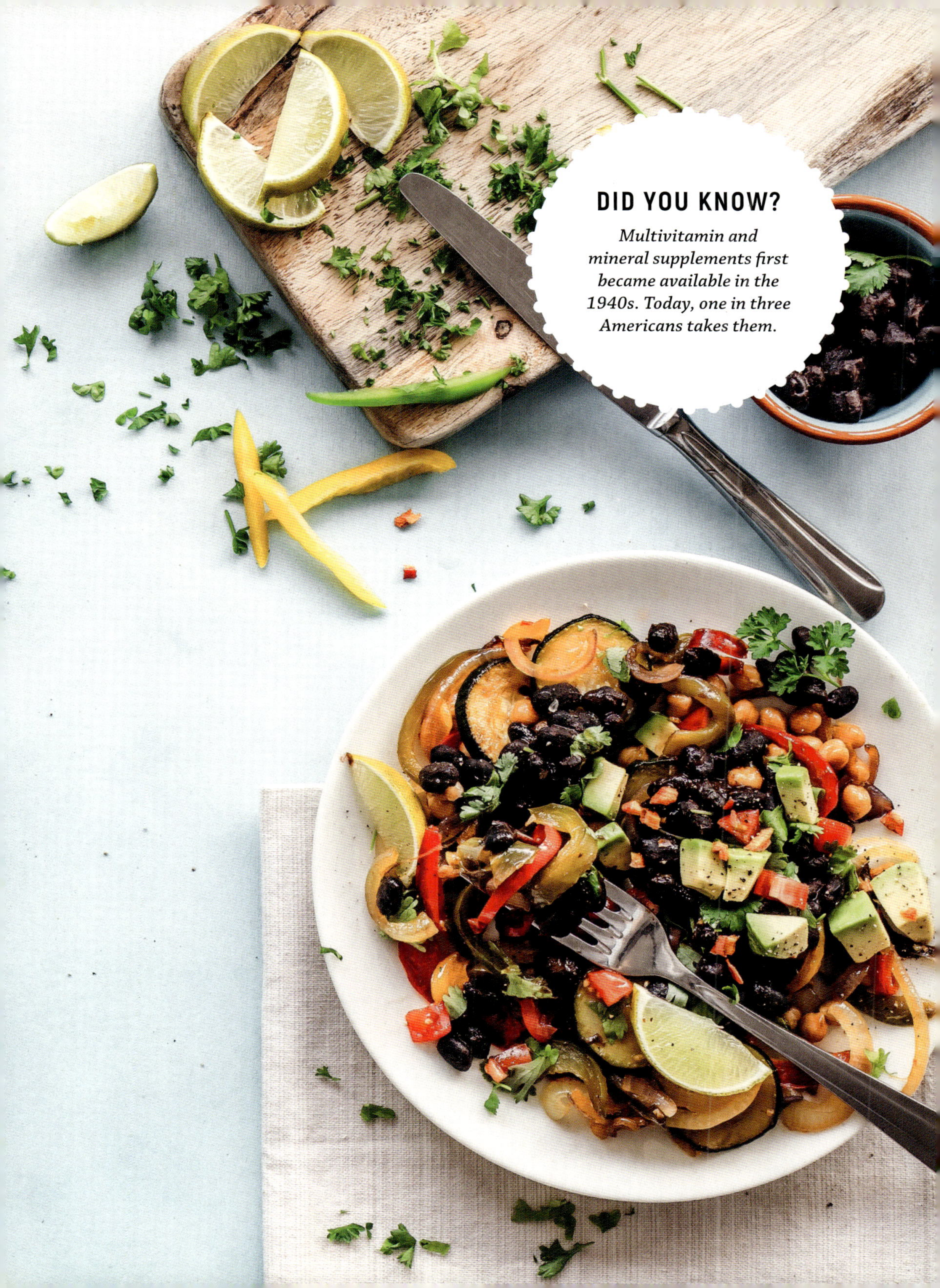

DID YOU KNOW?

Multivitamin and mineral supplements first became available in the 1940s. Today, one in three Americans takes them.

[VITAMINS AND MINERALS THAT WORK TOGETHER]

If you have already paged through the vitamins and minerals sections in this book, then you know that many of their roles are interconnected. Getting too much or too little of a certain nutrient can interfere with the functions of another, and deficiencies of several vitamins or minerals can occur simultaneously. Here are three of the best-known nutrient combos and how they work together to keep your body healthy.

VITAMIN D AND CALCIUM

There's a reason these two nutrients are always seen together in milk and dairy products. Without vitamin D, the body cannot properly regulate calcium. Vitamin D is responsible for signaling a series of events when blood calcium levels are too low. These include increasing the absorption of calcium from foods in the intestines, enhancing calcium reabsorption in the kidneys, and signaling the breakdown of bones to release calcium into the blood (see also pages 20 and 74).

Vitamin D deficiency therefore negatively impacts skeletal health. When there isn't enough vitamin D in the body to increase dietary calcium absorption, the body resorts to a more destructive way of maintaining calcium levels—taking it from the skeleton. In severe cases, this can lead to rickets in children and osteomalacia in adults. But even less overt cases of vitamin D deficiency may increase the risk of osteoporosis and other bone issues. To maintain adequate vitamin D and calcium levels, be sure to regularly incorporate foods from the lists on pages 19 and 73.

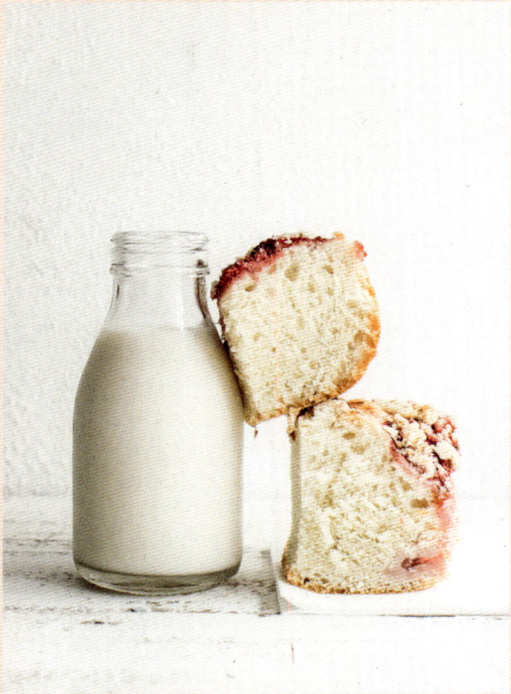

Drink milk that's been fortified with vitamin D to aid absorption of calcium.

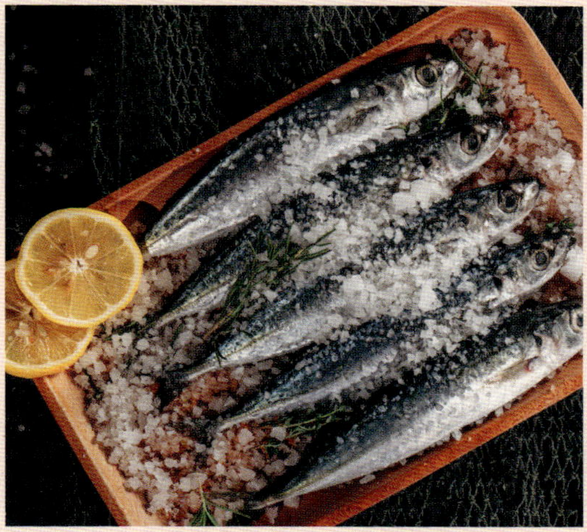

Serve fish baked or preserved in salt with a potassium-rich tomato salad on the side.

SODIUM AND POTASSIUM

Do you sometimes feel bloated and thirsty after eating salty foods? That's sodium at work in your body. The electrolytes all work together, and sodium and potassium in particular are very interconnected when it comes to maintaining blood pressure (see also pages 88 and 92).

When you eat a high volume of very salty foods, the body holds onto water to help maintain the right levels of sodium in the blood. This increases blood pressure. However, the effects of sodium can be counteracted by an adequate intake of potassium. Increasing consumption of potassium-rich foods can promote sodium excretion in the urine, which in turn helps lower blood pressure. Keeping sodium intake within the recommended daily limits while meeting potassium needs is key to maintaining healthy blood pressure.

VITAMIN B6, VITAMIN B12, AND FOLATE

The synchronous functions of folate and vitamins B6 and B12 may help protect against certain chronic diseases. These three vitamins work together to regulate levels of the amino acid homocysteine in the blood. When the body does not have adequate amounts of these vitamins, homocysteine may not be properly regulated and can accumulate in the blood. High levels of homocysteine have been linked to heart disease, dementia, stroke, and even osteoporosis. Getting enough B vitamins from foods may therefore be an important step in preventing these diseases.

However, studies offer mixed results on using supplements with B6, B12, and folate. Some research indicates that these supplements help reduce blood homocysteine levels, but this doesn't always translate into a reduced risk of disease. More research is needed. While the jury's still out, you should aim to eat a diet that's rich in B vitamins, which will help you feel energized and support the many other functions of these nutrients in the body.

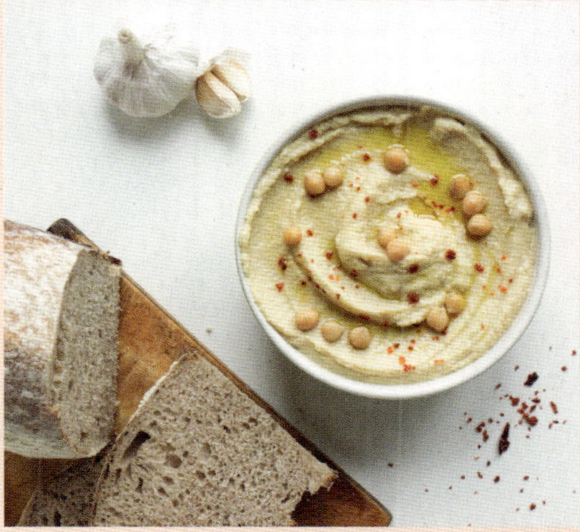

A serving of hummus will contribute to your vitamin B6 needs.

[EAT THE RAINBOW]

A plate full of colorful foods isn't just pretty. It's a good indication that you're eating loads of nutrients! Eating a rainbow of colors, instead of sticking to foods with the same hues, is a great way to get a variety of vitamins and minerals and to meet your daily needs.

The color of a food tells you a lot about its nutritional profile. In fact, some nutrients are responsible for the shades you see as you browse the farmers market or produce aisle. Beta-carotene, the provitamin A carotenoid discussed on page 15, is a red-orange pigment found in winter squashes, carrots, apricots, sweet potatoes, and cantaloupes. Additionally, foods with the same hue may have similar vitamin and mineral contents and contain the same types of other beneficial compounds.

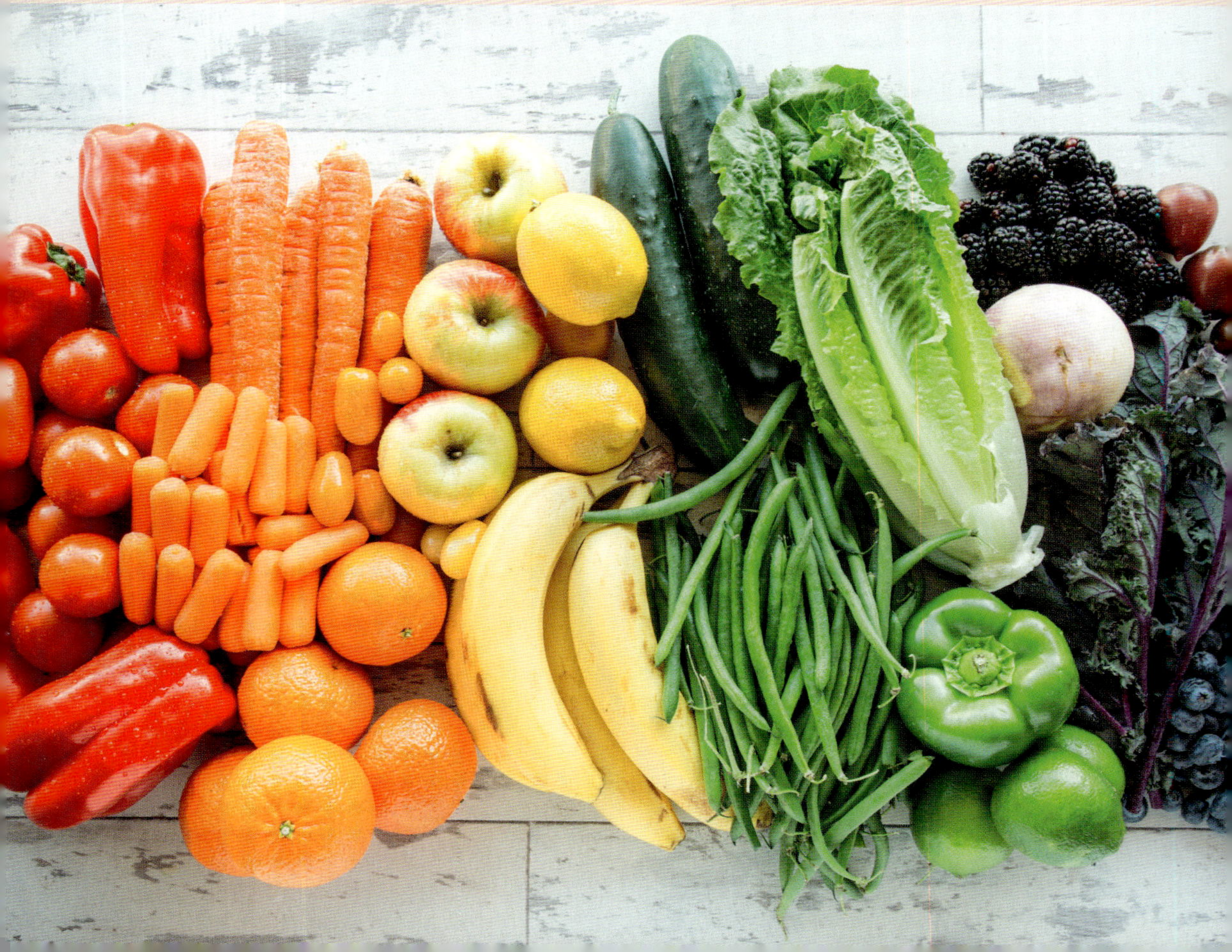

RED

Many of the listed foods are rich in vitamins A, C, and K, and also contain folate and potassium. Cranberries have some copper, radishes have riboflavin, and rhubarb carries vitamin K1.

Tomatoes, Beets, Radishes, Raspberries, Cranberries, Cherries, Chili peppers, Red bell peppers, Rhubarb, Watermelons, Pomegranates, Red kidney beans

ORANGE AND YELLOW

Some of the headliner orange and yellow plants, such as carrots and citrus, are loaded with vitamin C and beta-carotene, among many other nutrients. Pineapple provides manganese, while oranges contain calcium.

Carrots, Squashes, Oranges, Lemons, Persimmons, Mangoes, Sweet corn, Pineapples, Peaches, Cantaloupes

GREEN

Green veggies often contain folate, vitamins A, C, E, and K, magnesium, calcium, and iron. Mustard greens are a source of vitamin B6, and green grapes provide vitamin K1.

Spinach, Kale, Collard greens, Swiss chard, Mustard greens, Arugula, Bok choy, Broccoli, Brussels sprouts, Kiwis, Green lentils, Green apples, Green grapes, Asparagus, Lima beans, Broad beans, Green beans, Edamame, Peas

BLUE AND PURPLE

Fruits and veggies with these hues may have vitamins A and C, folate, choline, potassium, phosphorus, and copper. Eggplant has small amounts of manganese and niacin, while radicchio is rich in copper.

Purple cabbages, Eggplants, Blueberries, Figs, Purple cauliflowers, Plums, Purple carrots, Blackberries, Purple grapes, Radicchio

WHITE AND TAN

This group is the most varied, since many nuts, veggies, dairy products, grains, and beans have white or tan shades. Beans and grains provide zinc, iron, copper, and/or B vitamins, nuts and seeds have many of these nutrients plus magnesium and vitamin E, dairy products are rich in calcium and vitamin D, and white veggies offer selenium, vitamin C, and/or vitamin K.

White beans, Onions, Garlic, Chickpeas, Shallots, Black-eyed peas, Pinto beans, Brown rice, Parsnips, Quinoa, Almonds, Mushrooms, Sunflower seeds, Hazelnuts, Walnuts, Bananas, Cauliflowers, White apricots

HEALTHFUL PIGMENTS

There are many other colorful, health-promoting pigments found in fruits and veggies that aren't essential vitamins and minerals. Lycopene is a red pigment in tomatoes, watermelon, and papaya that boosts heart health. Betalains are the deep-red compounds responsible for the color and anti-inflammatory properties of beets. (They're also the reason your urine turns a harmless shade of pink after eating beets!) Anthocyanins, found in red, purple, and blue plants, such as cabbage, blueberries, cranberries, and eggplant, act as antioxidants.

DOs AND DON'Ts

- *DO eat at least one item from each color group every day if you can.*
- *DO vary the foods you choose from each group.*
- *DON'T stick to just one or two colors for the majority of your diet.*

[NUTRIENT-DENSE FOODS]

Even though it's common to refer to a food as a "good source" of specific nutrients, no foods contain just one nutrient. Instead, they provide a variety of vitamins and minerals. This list includes foods that are incredibly nutrient dense and that you can eat to increase your intake of several nutrients at once.

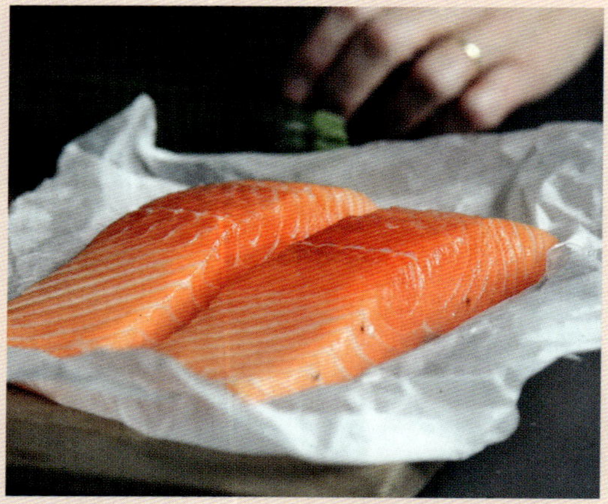

Lentils: Legumes offer many nutrients, and lentils are among the most nutritious. They're packed with folate and iron, in addition to phosphorus, copper, manganese, and thiamin.

Pumpkin seeds: Pumpkin seeds are small but mighty! They provide iron, zinc, calcium, magnesium, copper, and selenium.

Salmon: Salmon is one of the few dietary sources of vitamin D. It also packs good quantities of potassium, selenium, and B vitamins, including B12.

Eggs: Eggs are commonly referred to as one of the most nutritious foods on the planet, thanks to a high concentration of vitamins and minerals in both the yolk and white. They contain riboflavin, selenium, choline, biotin, and vitamins D and B12.

Organ meats: No list of nutrient-dense foods would be complete without mentioning liver and other organ meats. Beef liver in particular is an extremely concentrated source of nutrients, especially vitamins A and B12 and copper. If you don't have the stomach for liver, that's OK too, since you can still easily meet your nutrient needs without it.

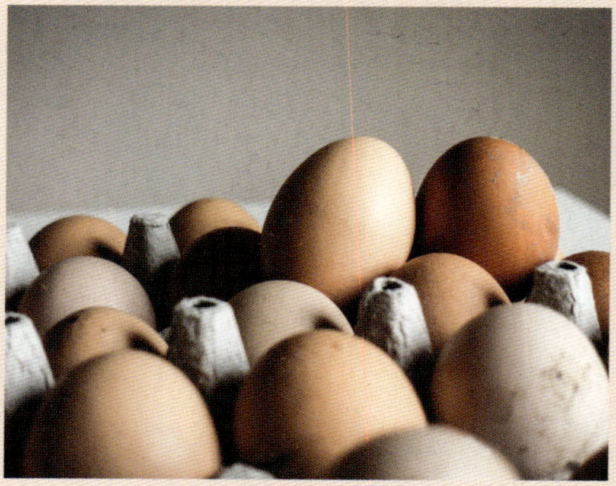

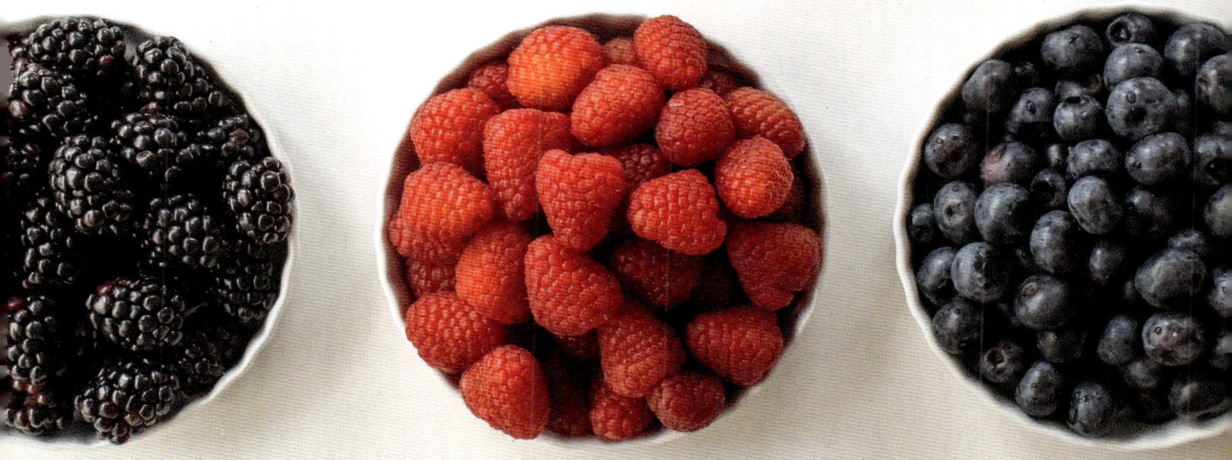

Potatoes: The humble spud gets a bad rap because of its high carb content, but potatoes are actually incredibly nutritious. Potatoes with their skin are loaded with potassium, copper, iron, magnesium, manganese, vitamin C, and B vitamins. Sweet potatoes contain many of these same nutrients, in addition to provitamin A carotenoids and vitamin E.

Broccoli: With high amounts of vitamins C and K, plus folate, potassium, and calcium, broccoli is a supremely nutritious vegetable.

Winter squashes: The brightly colored flesh of winter squashes indicates a high concentration of beta-carotene. Squashes also provide vitamin C, B vitamins, potassium, magnesium, iron, and manganese. Different types of winter squashes are listed as good sources of certain nutrients throughout this book. In most cases, you can assume that other types of winter squashes provide similar amounts of a certain nutrient, such as vitamins A or C, potassium, and magnesium.

Berries: Strawberries, blackberries, blueberries, and raspberries all provide tons of micronutrients. Strawberries are rich in vitamin C, folate, and potassium; blueberries and blackberries provide vitamins C and K and manganese; and raspberries contain many of these nutrients as well as biotin.

IS TAKING MULTIVITAMINS WORTH IT?

Studies offer weak and conflicting evidence for the possible benefits of taking multivitamins, and getting nutrients from a varied diet with nutritious foods appears to be better than taking pills. If you have deficiencies, supplementing with specific nutrients under the recommendations of a health care provider is usually recommended. They may be beneficial for people on special diets, older adults, and pregnant or breastfeeding women. While the amounts of nutrients typically found in multivitamins are unlikely to cause harm and may help fill a nutrient gap in your diet, there's not much evidence for their benefits.

[ANTIOXIDANTS]

You've likely seen the term "antioxidants" on food packaging, supplements, beauty creams, and many other products. There are even sodas, energy drinks, and snack bars that boast their antioxidant content. Many people think of antioxidants as disease-fighting compounds of which you must increase your intake. But is all the hype really warranted?

ALL ABOUT ANTIOXIDANTS

Antioxidants are compounds that protect the body from oxidative damage caused by reactive molecules called free radicals. Free radicals aren't all bad, and they're actually necessary for certain functions in the body. But when too many free radicals form, as a result of exposure to air pollution, cigarette smoke, alcohol, certain drugs, UV rays, or fried foods, the body enters a state of oxidative stress. In this state, free radicals outnumber antioxidants. The resulting damage to the body over time can increase the risk of heart disease, certain cancers, and diabetes.

The body has its own antioxidant system to protect against free radicals, but you can also get antioxidants from foods. Vitamins C and E, beta-carotene (a provitamin A carotenoid), selenium, copper, and zinc have antioxidant properties, and it's thought that foods rich in these nutrients protect against disease. Other carotenoids, including lycopene, lutein, and zeaxanthin, as well as anthocyanins, flavanols, quercetin, and catechins are compounds in foods that may also act as antioxidants. But keep in mind that each one has unique roles in the body, and antioxidants work in combination with other nutrients and compounds in foods. Taking antioxidants alone in supplement form, or consuming products with high amounts of an isolated nutrient, won't have the same effect.

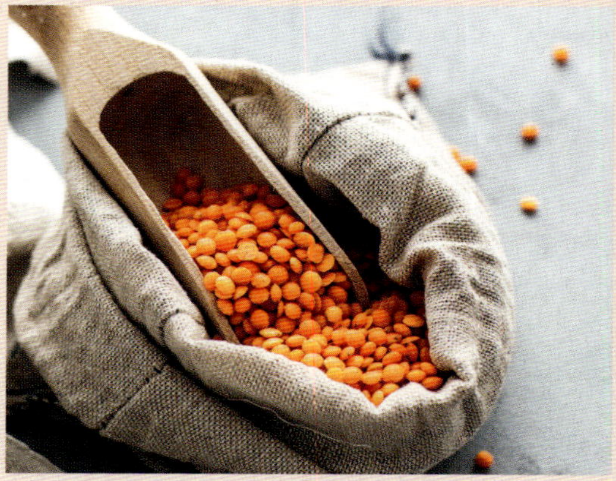

Red lentils are a source of selenium and beta-carotene.

In short, it's best to get nutrients with antioxidant activity by eating a variety of foods, not supplements. Research has shown that higher intakes of antioxidant-rich fruits, vegetables, and legumes are linked to better health, longevity, and a lower risk of disease. But studies that look at the effects of antioxidant supplements offer little support for the idea that they have the same benefits. In fact, high supplemental doses of antioxidants may actually be harmful and are not recommended outside of medical supervision.

BOOSTING ANTIOXIDANT INTAKE NATURALLY

With so many great food sources of naturally occurring antioxidants, there's no need to waste your money on expensive supplements and products. Here are some of the best antioxidant-rich foods to enjoy!

- **Vitamin C:** Oranges, grapefruits, kiwis, papayas, and broccoli contain vitamin C.
- **Vitamin E:** Olive oil, avocados, wheat germ, and sunflower seeds all contain vitamin E.
- **Beta-carotene:** Cantaloupes, and many types of winter squashes (butternut, acorn, and kabocha) contain beta-carotene.
- **Selenium:** Brazil nuts, shrimp, turkey, and lentils are all good sources.
- **Copper:** Oysters, shiitake mushrooms, and cashew nuts are all good sources.
- **Zinc:** Shellfish—oysters, crab, and lobster are all good sources.
- **Lycopene:** Tomatoes and watermelons are sources of this carotenoid.
- **Lutein and zeaxanthin:** Green leafy vegetables and egg yolks are sources of these carotenoids.
- **Quercetin:** Onions are loaded with this.

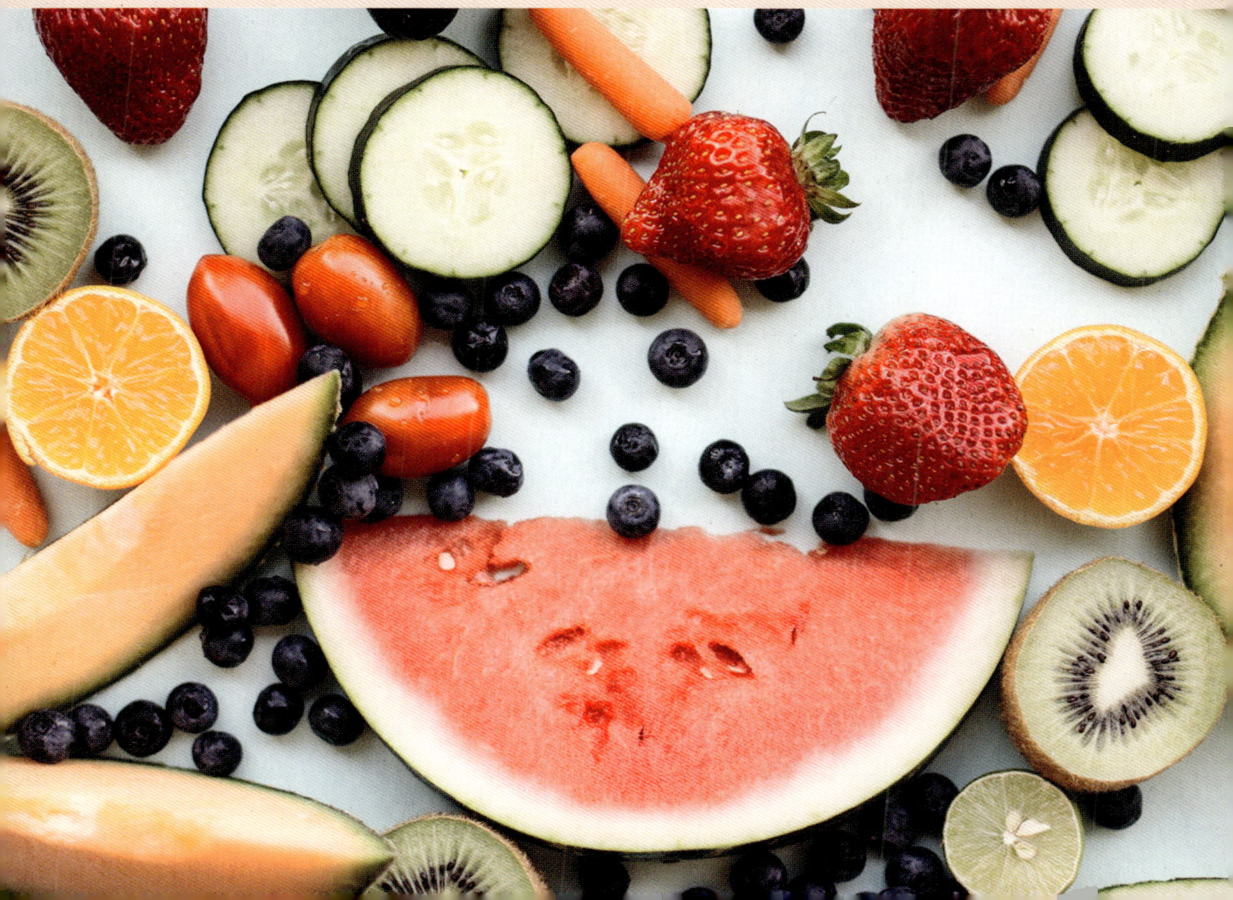

[BEYOND VITAMINS]

Even though this is a book about vitamins and minerals, several other supplements are worth mentioning. The previous sections have already established that, except when there's a specific reason to take a supplement, it's almost always better to meet nutrient needs through foods and not pills. But what about supplements that aren't vitamins and minerals, such as omega-3s, melatonin, and St. John's wort?

Here's a glossary of commonly available supplements and what the research has to say about each of them. Always speak with a health care provider before trying any new supplements to confirm that they will be safe and beneficial for you.

OMEGA-3 FATTY ACIDS

Fish oil is an excellent source of omega-3 fatty acids, an essential nutrient that makes up cell membranes, exhibits anti-inflammatory effects in the body, and is necessary for healthy neurological development. Current recommendations suggest eating fatty fish twice a week to meet omega-3 needs, but many people fall short and don't get enough of these fatty acids. Plant-based sources include walnuts, chia seeds, and flaxseeds, but omega-3s from these foods are generally not as well absorbed as those from fish.

Inadequate omega-3 intake may contribute to cognitive deterioration, neuropsychiatric disorders, heart disease, and other issues. However, it's unclear if fish oil supplementation can help prevent or manage these conditions. The most promising effects of supplementation appear to be related to heart disease. Some studies suggest that omega-3 supplements are helpful in reducing high triglyceride levels and death from heart disease, while other research indicates that it's not yet clear whether supplements help with issues like cognitive decline. At the end of the day, fish oil supplements are usually not necessary for generally healthy people with a low heart disease risk and a balanced diet that includes fish and/or plant-based sources of omega-3.

ADAPTOGENS

As their name suggests, adaptogens are herbs that help the body "adapt" to stress and reduce exhaustion. Studies back their proposed effects, from ashwagandha's ability to reduce stress to the memory-boosting effects of American ginseng. Other adaptogens include goji berry, licorice root, tulsi (holy basil), rhodiola, and astragalus. Each one has unique effects; some may energize you, while others calm you down. They are thought to be generally safe, but should only be taken in proper dosages and for short periods of time. There is also concern of medication interaction with some adaptogens. Depending on your needs, they may be worth exploring, but only after you've done your research and contacted your health care provider.

FLAVONOIDS

These compounds are found in vegetables, fruits, tea, wine, coffee, and chocolate. They exhibit antioxidant effects in the body, and consumption of flavonoids from foods has been linked to heart benefits, a lower risk of type 2 diabetes, and anticancer effects. But similar to antioxidants (see pages 140–41), flavonoid supplements likely don't offer the same benefits as flavonoid-rich foods. Stick to eating a variety of plant foods to reap their benefits.

PROBIOTICS

Probiotics refer to healthy bacteria that reside in your gut and promote optimal digestion and health. There are many unique strains of probiotics that may address different health conditions. An imbalance in gut bacteria, that occurs when "good" probiotics are outnumbered by less friendly organisms, may be linked to obesity, type 2 diabetes, heart disease, colorectal cancer, and even depression. However, research that supports the use of probiotic supplements to address these conditions is still limited. If you have a specific concern and want to try out a probiotic, discuss with your health care provider to see which strain may be best for you. Otherwise, healthy adults can get plenty of probiotics from foods such as yogurt, kefir, kimchi, and kombucha.

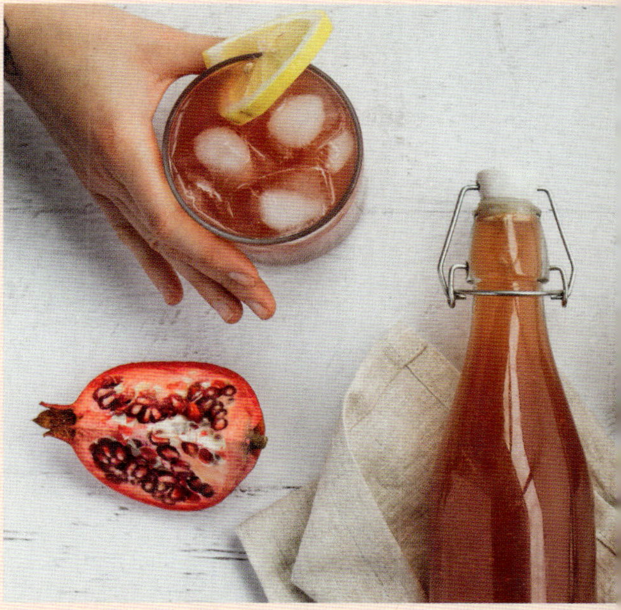

Pomegranate-infused kombucha.

MELATONIN

Melatonin is a hormone that helps you fall asleep. The body naturally produces melatonin, but it's also commonly taken as a supplement. Current research suggests that melatonin supplements can help people with sleep disorders fall asleep easier and also reduce jet lag. Melatonin is generally considered safe. If you are interested in trying it, consult with your health care provider, especially if you are taking medications for other health conditions. Look for reputable brands that have been tested for quality by a third party and follow package instructions closely for appropriate dosing.

CHECK THE LABEL

The FDA does not regulate supplements as tightly as medications, and supplements on the market do not need to be tested for purity, safety, or effectiveness. When choosing supplements, look for brands that have been tested by a third party to make sure you are getting a high-quality product. This type of testing is usually indicated on a supplement's label and may be represented by a logo from NSF International, NSF Certified for Sport, United States Pharmacopeia (USP), Informed-Choice, ConsumerLab, or the Banned Substances Control Group (BSCG).

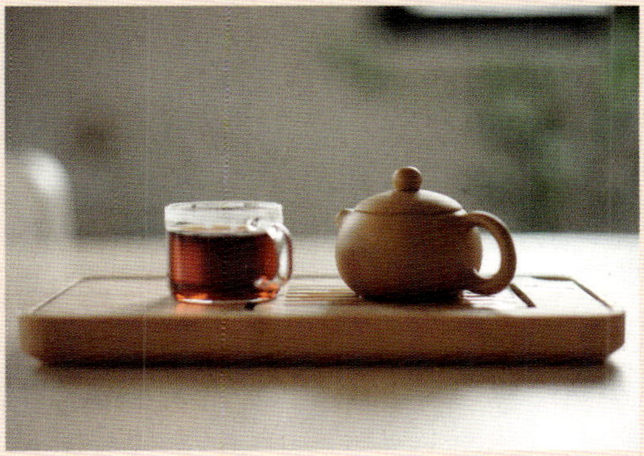

All black and green teas are good sources of naturally occuring flavonoids.

COLLAGEN

Collagen is the most abundant protein in the body and gives structure to skin, bones, connective tissue, and cartilage that cushions joints. Due to these roles in the body, collagen supplements are thought to lead to smooth skin, stronger muscles, increased bone mass, and improvements in joint pain or arthritis.

While some studies support the supposed benefits of taking collagen supplements or increasing collagen consumption via bone broth, poultry skin, or gelatin, there's still debate about how collagen acts in the body once consumed. Collagen, like other proteins, gets broken down into amino acids that the body then reassembles into proteins it needs. Thus, consuming collagen from supplements doesn't necessarily mean your body's collagen levels will increase. If you are interested in trying collagen for a period of time to see if it benefits you, current research suggests that collagen supplements are generally safe. The most common form is collagen peptide powder, which can be mixed in to drinks, soups, and other recipes.

COENZYME Q10

Coenzyme Q10 (CoQ10) is a compound found in the mitochondria of cells that helps with cellular energy generation and acts as an antioxidant. The body produces CoQ10, but production decreases with age. People with diabetes, heart disease, and some cancers may have low levels of CoQ10, but it's not clear if CoQ10 deficiency causes certain health issues or develops as a result of them.

Supplementing with CoQ10 may improve blood sugar regulation in those with type 2 diabetes, decrease the number and severity of migraines, reduce inflammation associated with asthma, and improve exercise performance. CoQ10 supplements may also help with fertility by improving sperm and egg quality. The best-absorbed supplemental form of CoQ10 is ubiquinol, but CoQ10 from foods like organ meats, fatty fish, oranges, strawberries, cauliflower, and lentils is also well absorbed. CoQ10 supplements are well tolerated and appear to be very safe, with almost no reported side effects from available research. Still, it's important to purchase them from a reputable company.

TOPICAL VS. ORAL SUPPLEMENTS

Some supplements have different effects when applied topically compared to when they're taken as pills. CoQ10, vitamin C, and collagen are often found in facial lotions aimed at reducing wrinkles and improving skin appearance. Research on the effects of these products is limited, but dermatologists note that the skin cannot absorb collagen. If using collagen has any benefits for the skin, it would most likely result from taking pills rather than using creams. Whether or not CoQ10 or vitamin C serums work is still being investigated, but some studies suggest they may improve skin appearance over time.

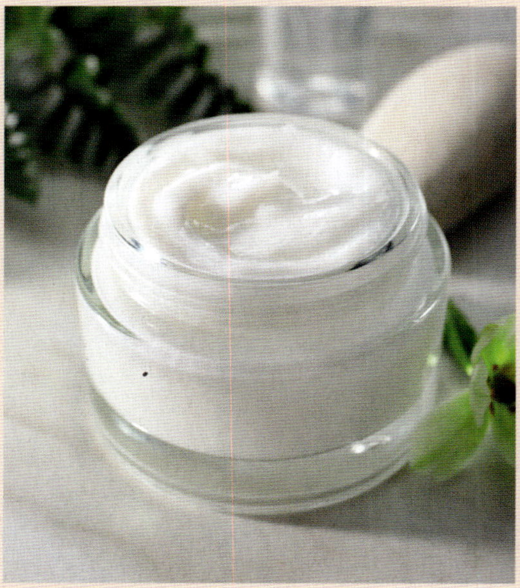

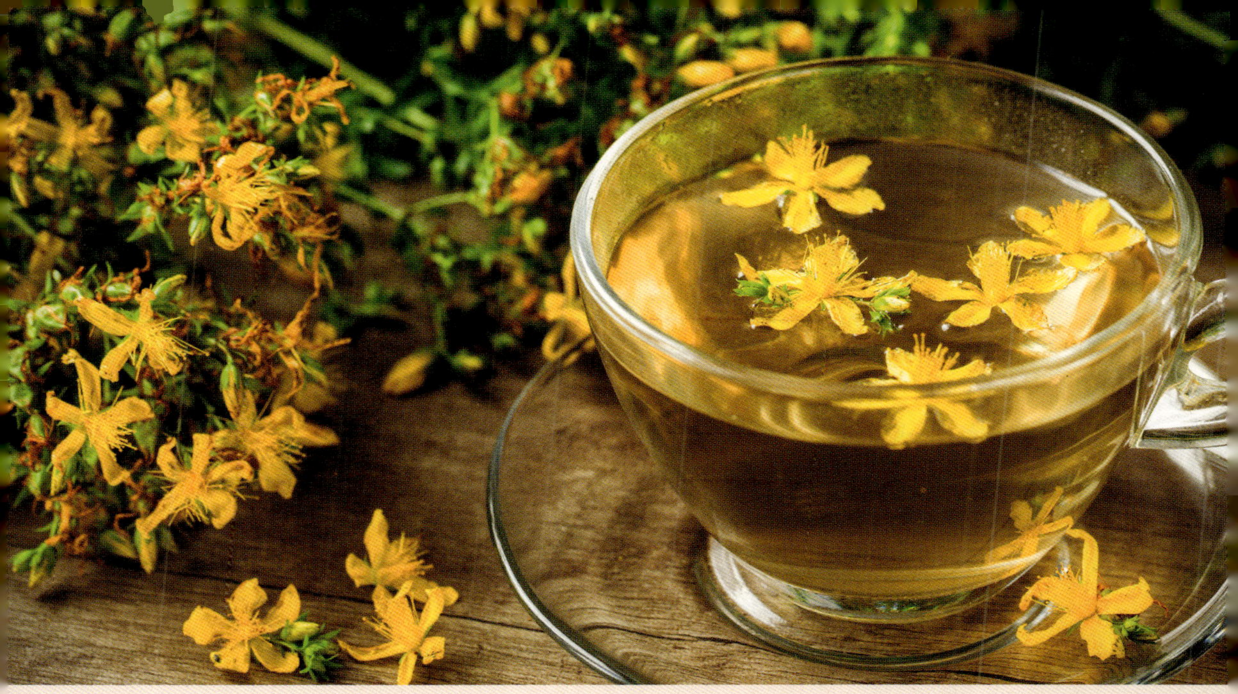

RED YEAST RICE EXTRACT

Red yeast rice, a type of fermented rice, is considered one of the best "natural" therapies for high cholesterol levels. This is because it contains the compound monacolin K, which is the same active ingredient in the cholesterol-lowering medication lovastatin. Scientific trials have found that red yeast rice supplements can lower total and "bad" LDL cholesterol levels. However, the range of monacolin K in red yeast products may vary widely. The FDA has also banned the sale of supplements that have enough of the ingredient to make them comparable to lovastatin, since they have not undergone the same degree of approval process as drugs. Red yeast rice may have similar side effects as prescription statins, such as bloating and gas, liver damage, and muscle injury. Even more, a 2014 analysis of red yeast rice supplements found that some products may contain a compound that forms during the culturing of red yeast rice and can cause kidney damage. Due to the lack of regulation and potential side effects, it's vital to speak to your health care provider before trying red yeast rice in place of or in addition to prescription, cholesterol-lowering medications.

ST. JOHN'S WORT

Derived from a yellow flowering shrub, St. John's wort is most commonly used as a supplement to treat depression. A fairly substantial body of research suggests that it may be as effective as pharmaceutical anti-depressant medications for mild to moderate depression, but keep in mind that it is not recommended in addition to pharmaceutical antidepressants.

St. John's wort can interfere with several medications, making them less effective and/or resulting in dangerous side effects. These include antidepressants, anxiety medications like Xanax, HIV drugs, birth control pills, blood thinners, statins, organ transplant medications, and anti-seizure medications. Since the FDA does not regulate St. John's wort in the same way as medications, there may be a wide variability in the contents and purity of available supplements that contain it. Discuss with your health care provider before trying St. John's wort, especially if you are taking other medications.

[NUTRITION AND HEALTH ISSUES]

The familiar saying "food is medicine" illuminates the powerful role of nutrition in health and disease. Poor nutrition can increase the risk of many chronic diseases, including hypertension, type 2 diabetes, and heart disease, while good nutrition can help prevent and manage these conditions. If you are living with a chronic disease that can be improved via dietary changes, consider working with a registered dietitian (RD/RDN). A dietitian will assess your diet and recommend practical tips for managing your health condition.

In this section, you will read about the vitamins and minerals of concern and importance for specific conditions to give you an idea of how micronutrients play a role in the nutritional management of disease. But remember, this section offers a brief overview. Your dietitian and other health care providers can create much more personalized recommendations that cover many aspects of diet and lifestyle in addition to vitamins and minerals.

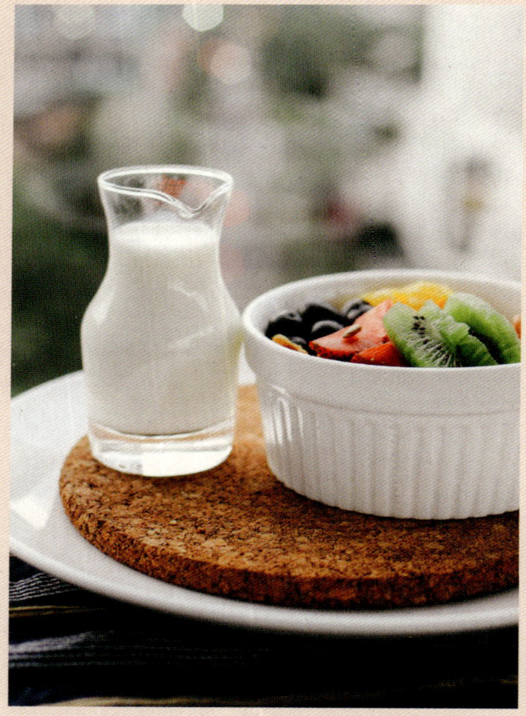

People with osteoporosis can benefit from drinking vitamin D fortified milk.

HYPERTENSION

As discussed on pages 87 and 91, two of the main dietary interventions for high blood pressure are decreasing sodium intake while increasing consumption of potassium-rich foods. Check out the tips on page 92 for cutting back on your sodium intake. To up your potassium consumption, review the list on page 87 to identify which foods are good sources of this nutrient.

INFLAMMATORY BOWEL DISEASE (IBD)

Individuals with Crohn's disease or ulcerative colitis are at a higher risk for micronutrient deficiencies, due to malabsorption, insufficient intake, and/or increased losses. Micronutrients of concern include calcium, vitamin D, vitamin B12, iron, zinc, and magnesium. Depending on the assessment and recommendations of their health care providers, individuals with IBD may need to increase intake of and/or supplement with certain vitamins and/or minerals.

KIDNEY DISEASE

Individuals with advanced kidney disease need to watch their consumption of certain micronutrients, especially potassium and phosphorus. Impaired kidney function makes it harder for the body to get rid of these nutrients, which can lead to high blood levels and dangerous symptoms. Some straightforward, high to low potassium food swaps include raisins to dried cranberries, spinach to green beans, and mashed potatoes to mashed cauliflower. Additionally, be cognizant of your consumption of these high-phosphorus foods: yogurt, milk, dairy products, dark-colored sodas, nuts, and bran cereals.

OSTEOPOROSIS

It's well known that calcium and vitamin D are important nutrients for bone health, but magnesium, potassium, and vitamins C and K also help keep bones strong. If you have osteoporosis, aim to eat a balanced diet with a variety of food sources that provide these nutrients. Fortified dairy products are a good source of calcium and vitamin D, while almonds, bok choy, collard greens, and chia seeds provide plant-based calcium. Prunes (dried plums) are another bone-building food, providing potassium and magnesium, while broccoli is a good source of vitamins C and K.

Leafy greens, such as bok choy, can help boost vitamin K intake in the diet

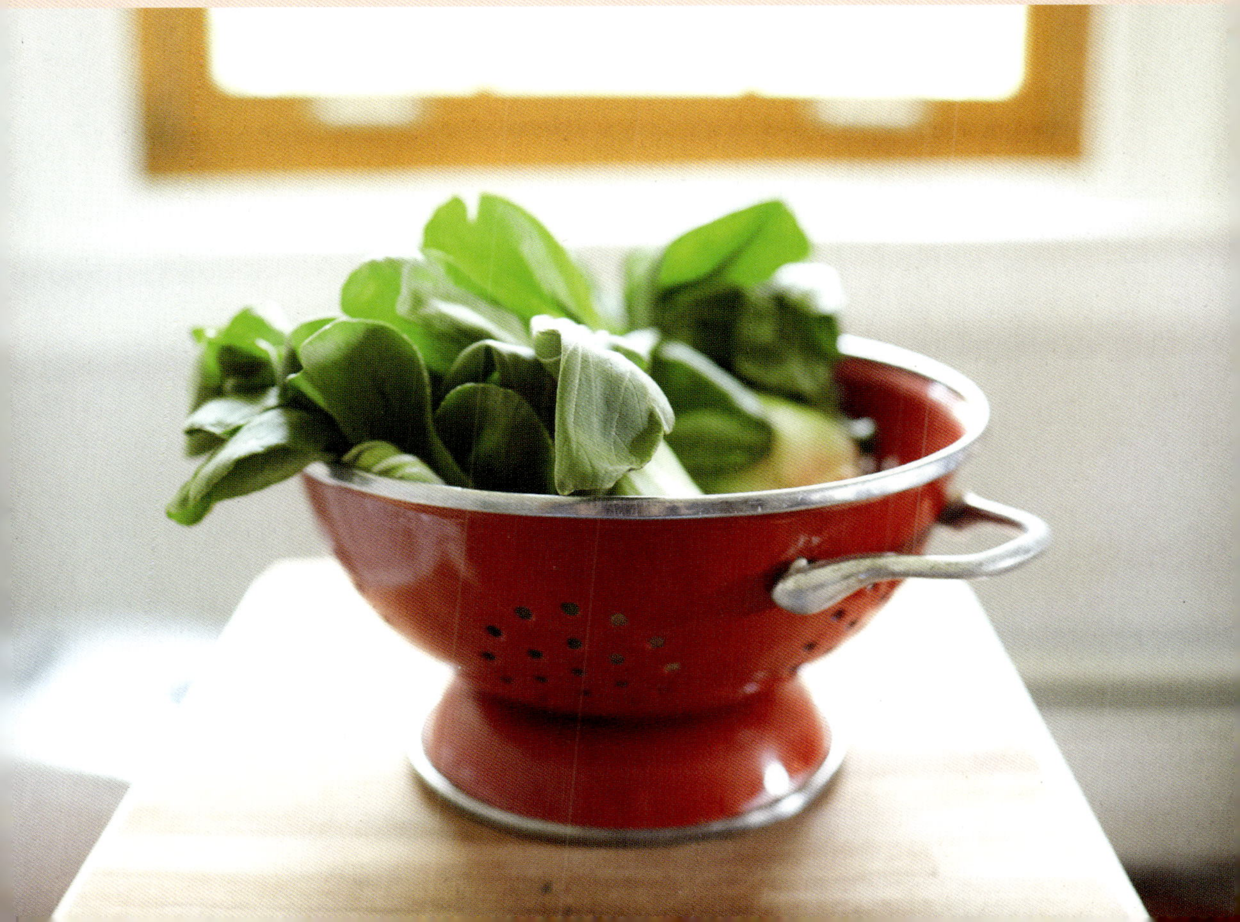

[SPECIAL DIETS]

If you follow a special diet for personal and/or health reasons, you may need to pay more attention to meeting the recommended intakes for certain nutrients. Eating patterns that restrict entire food groups can make it challenging to get enough vitamins and minerals. Here are some common diets and nutrients of concern for each one.

VEGETARIAN AND VEGAN

Lacto-ovo vegetarians who eat eggs and dairy products usually do not have a problem meeting their nutrient needs. Vegetarians who eat few animal products, as well as vegans who avoid all animal foods, may be more prone to nutrient deficiencies. A vegetarian or vegan diet that does not incorporate a variety of foods, including fortified products, may increase the likelihood of deficiencies of vitamins B12 and D, iron, zinc, and calcium.

As discussed on pages 113 and 129, iron and zinc from plants are generally not as well absorbed as animal-based sources of these nutrients. Plus, vitamin B12 only exists naturally in animal foods, so it's important to get enough of this nutrient from fortified plant foods or supplements. Fortunately, there are many vegan-friendly supplements of vitamin B12 and other nutrients available.

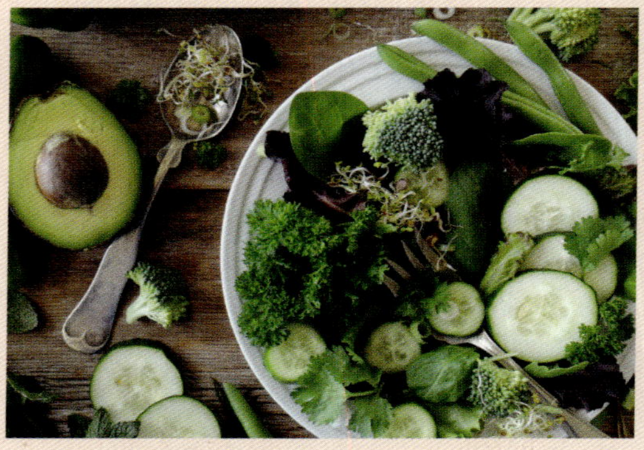

A vegetarian salad of raw green veggies.

KETOGENIC DIET

The low-carb, high-fat keto diet typically restricts or severely limits starchy vegetables, most fruits, beans, whole grains, and some dairy products such as milk and yogurt. These restrictions can lead to inadequate intakes of certain nutrients, including calcium, vitamins C, D, and E, magnesium, phosphorus, potassium, sodium, and some B vitamins. It's important to consult with a health care provider before trying the keto diet and to consider working with a dietitian to plan meals that minimize the risk of nutrient deficiencies.

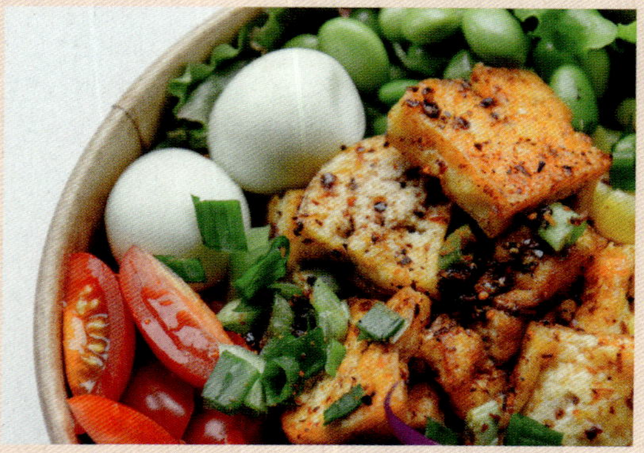

A low-carb ketogenic meal.

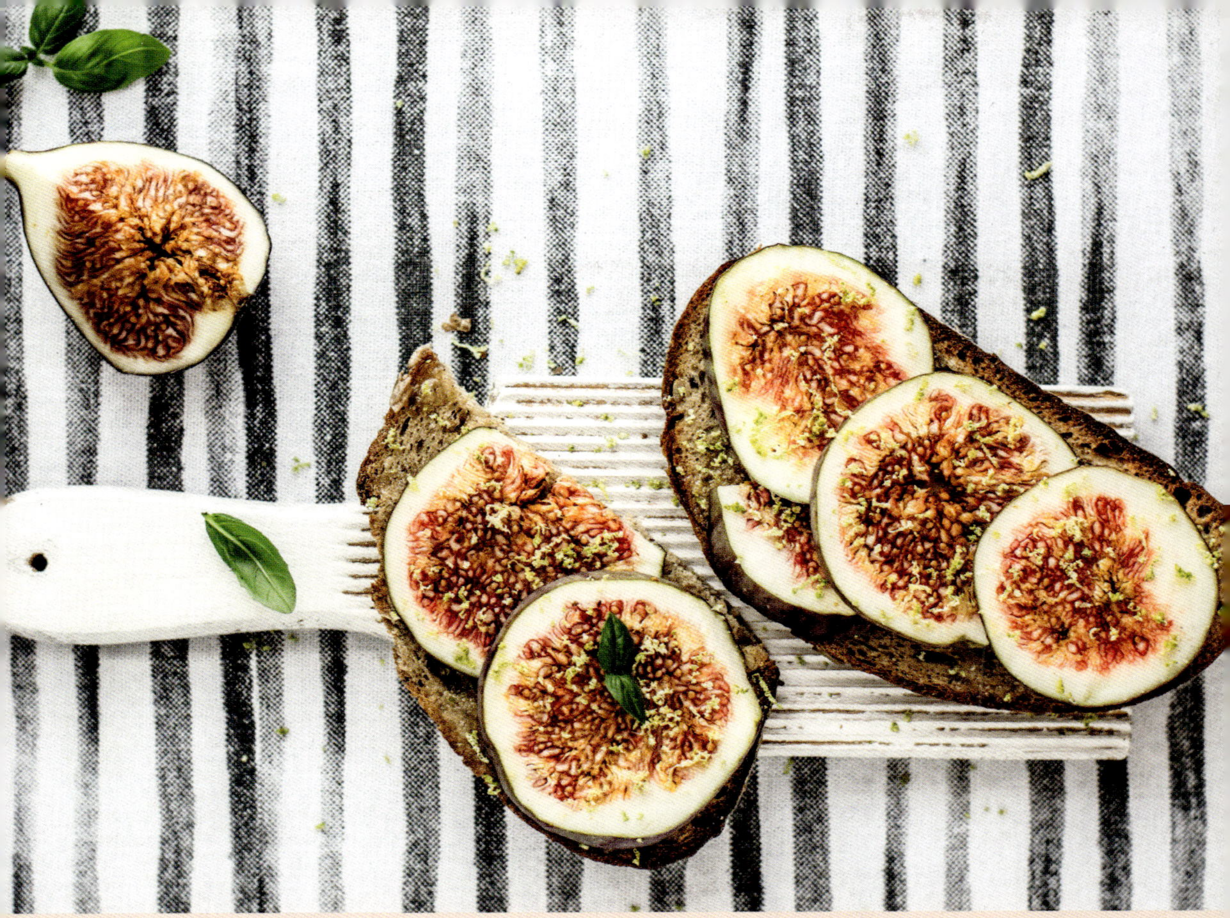

Figs are among the alternatives to dairy products when it comes to sources of calcium.

DAIRY-FREE

Milk and dairy products are some of the best sources of calcium and vitamin D in the diet. So, avoiding dairy products while also eating a diet that lacks variety may put you at risk of not getting enough of these important nutrients. To ensure adequate nutritional intake on a dairy-free diet, include plant-based foods that have been fortified with vitamin D, such as orange juice and nut milks, fatty fish, and egg yolks. Leafy greens, almonds, figs, chia seeds, and tofu made with calcium sulfate are good non-dairy sources of calcium.

GLUTEN-FREE

Individuals with celiac disease or gluten intolerance may suffer from nutritional deficiencies due to inadequate intake and poor absorption. Gluten-containing grain products are often enriched with vitamins and minerals, while most of their gluten-free counterparts are not. In addition, those who need to eat a gluten-free diet may not include enough variety to get adequate amounts of vitamins and minerals. Common nutrient deficiencies on a gluten-free diet include B vitamins (thiamin, riboflavin, niacin, and folate), iron, calcium, zinc, magnesium, and vitamins B12 and D.

[NUTRITION BY THE SEASON]

Fresh snow falling, spring flowers blooming, daylight stretching into evening, and leaves changing colors are quintessential markers of the four seasons. These transitions from season to season also mark a change in the body's nutritional needs. Depending on geographic location, you may need to be warier of getting certain nutrients at different times of the year. In some cases, foods that are in season during a particular period also tend to be some of the best sources of nutrients that the body needs.

Here is a helpful guide for maintaining good nutrition during the changing seasons. Keep in mind that if you live in a temperate area with plenty of sunshine and mild seasonal changes, these tips may not apply to you as much as they do to individuals in colder regions who experience all four seasons.

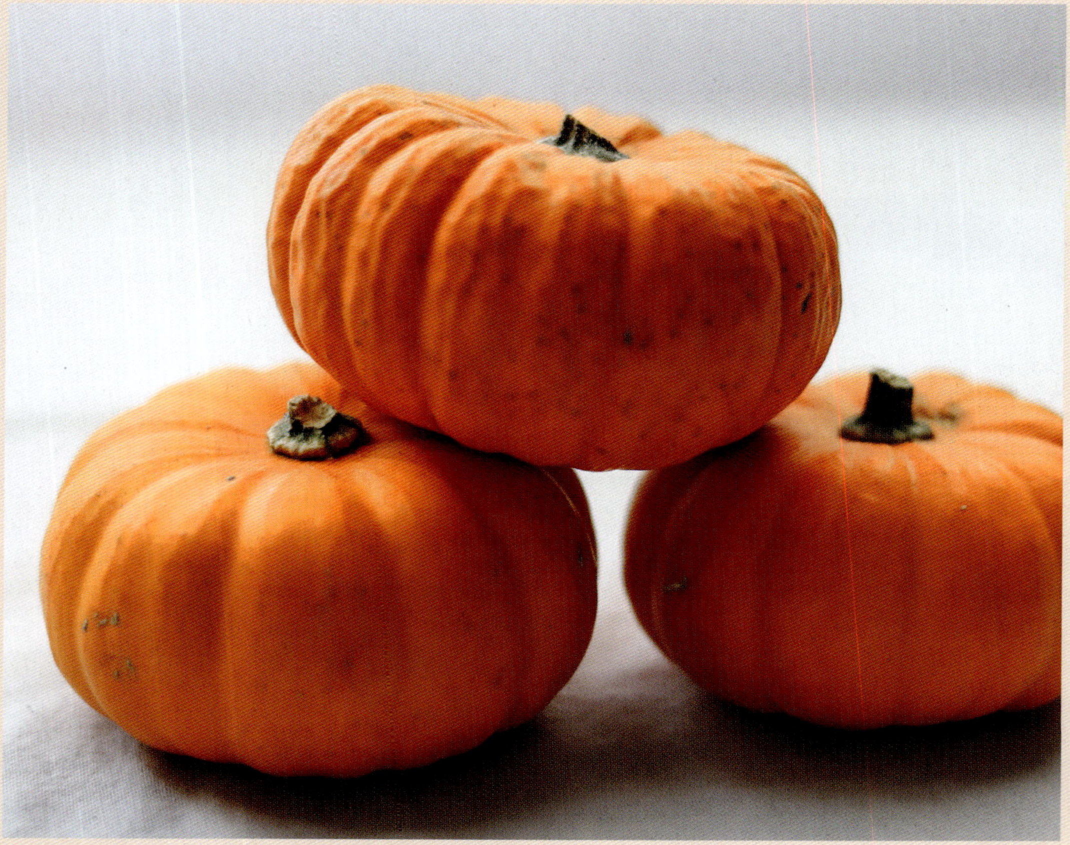

FALL AND WINTER

If you live in areas above a latitude of 37 degrees north (you can find this by tracing a line across North America from Virginia Beach to San Jose), the amount of sunlight from November through March is not sufficient for your body to produce enough vitamin D.

Since not getting enough vitamin D during the winter may negatively impact immunity during cold and flu season, it's important to increase intake of fortified foods and fatty fish. Other important nutrients for maintaining immune health include vitamins C and E, selenium, beta-carotene, and zinc. While it's not necessary to take supplements or drastically increase your intake of these nutrients, it is important to eat a diet that includes a variety of foods that provide them. Squashes that are in season during the fall and winter, including pumpkin, butternut, acorn, delicata, and kabocha, are some of the richest sources of beta-carotene and vitamin C. The brightly colored flesh of these veggies isn't the only part that will keep you healthy in the cold weather. Pumpkin and squash seeds also contain significant amounts of zinc, a vital nutrient for immunity.

SPOTLIGHT ON VITAMIN D

Some experts worry that the buzz surrounding vitamin D has led people to supplement with this nutrient unnecessarily. The number of Americans taking vitamin D supplements increased by 590% between 1999 and 2014. The debate continues about whether vitamin D deficiency is as prevalent as some people think it is and if supplements are actually beneficial for healthy individuals without true deficiency. Some research even suggests that while vitamin D supplements may correct deficiency, they don't improve the issues associated with low levels of this nutrient, such as increased fracture risk or poor mood. Finally, excess vitamin D from supplements can cause high blood calcium levels, which leads to nausea and vomiting, constipation, diarrhea, fatigue, and frequent urination.

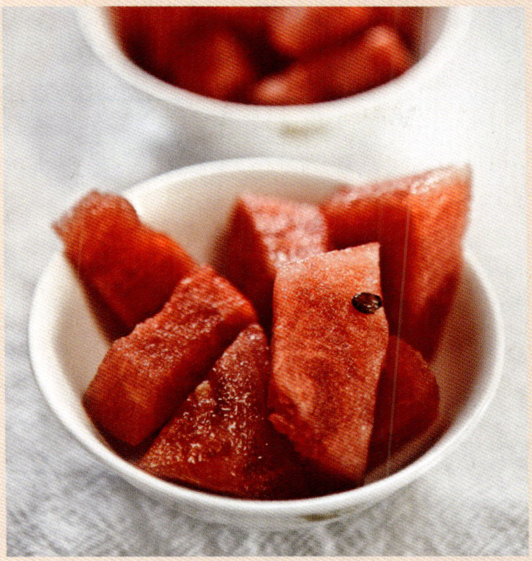

SPRING AND SUMMER

Spring is often considered a time of rejuvenation, and it presents an opportunity to freshen up your meals and enjoy some new foods. As the days get longer and schedules fill up with commitments, spring foods offer the energizing nutrients you need.

Vegetables that are abundant in the spring, including leafy greens, peas, and artichokes, offer B vitamins that support energy-yielding processes in the body. Once summer begins and temperatures increase, you may begin to sweat more and need more fluids. Fortunately, fruits and veggies that are in season during the summer have high water contents that can count toward your daily fluid intake. These include cucumbers, watermelon, zucchini, and tomatoes. The summer is also a time to get out in the sun to boost vitamin D levels. Aim for 10 to 30 minutes of sun on bare skin, preferably around midday, a few days per week during April through October. However, remember to take appropriate precautions if you have fair skin or are at increased risk of skin cancer.

[NUTRIENTS THROUGH THE LIFE CYCLE]

All humans need the same nutrients for life. These include the essential amino acids and fatty acids, carbohydrates, and the vitamins and minerals included in this book. But as you may have noticed as you read through Parts One and Two, some stages of the life cycle require different quantities of the essential nutrients.

Nutrient needs increase during pregnancy and lactation, infants and children often need more nutrients relative to body size than adults, and elderly individuals should get more of certain vitamins and minerals. Here's an overview of nutritional requirements through the life cycle.

PREGNANCY

Expectant mothers need more calories to support a growing baby, but they also require more of certain vitamins and minerals.

Nutrients of concern: Pregnant women need more folate, a vitamin that is essential for rapid cell division and the development of the baby's brain and spinal cord. Folate deficiency during pregnancy has been linked to neural tube defects and poor birth outcomes. Prenatal vitamins contain supplemental forms of folate—folic acid or methylfolate—to help women meet their increased needs. (See page 51 for folate-rich foods to include during pregnancy.)

Iron needs increase to 27 mg per day during pregnancy. More iron is necessary for the blood to transport oxygen to the growing baby. It's also highly important to meet needs for calcium, zinc, and vitamins C and D during pregnancy. Teenage mothers need more calcium to support both the baby and their own developing skeletons. Individuals who follow diets that restrict certain foods, such as vegan or vegetarian eating patterns, may need additional supplements. Women should always follow medical advice about foods to avoid during pregnancy.

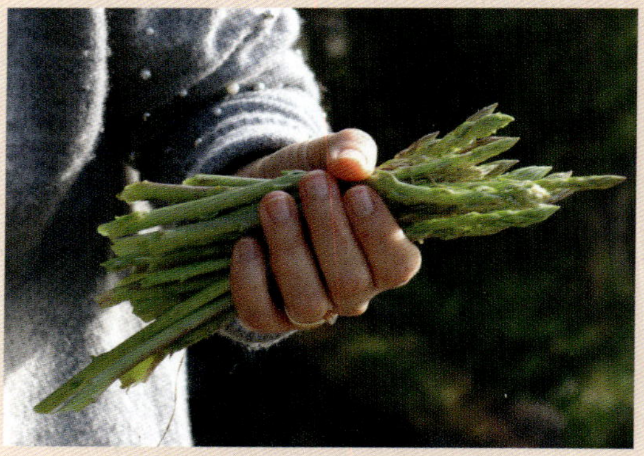

Asparagus is a good source of folate (vitamin B9).

LACTATION

Breastfeeding requires more calories, and lactating mothers should aim to eat a varied, nutritious diet to support the growth of their babies via breast milk.

Nutrients of concern: It's recommended that breastfeeding moms take a multivitamin or continue with their prenatal vitamin. Moms who eat a vegan or vegetarian diet may need more vitamin B12 from supplements. Women who don't get enough vitamin D from sun exposure or diet may need additional supplemental vitamin D.

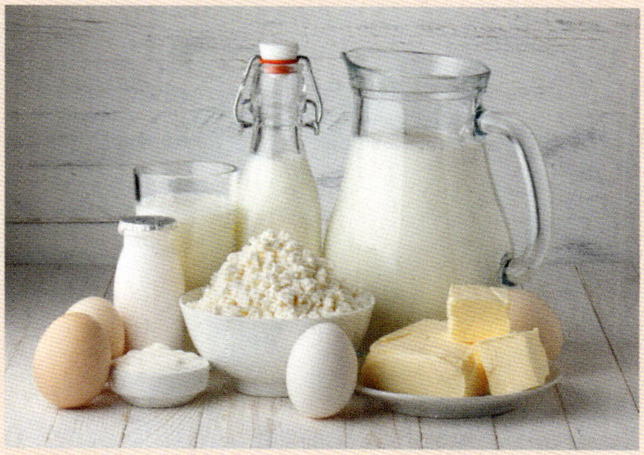

Growing children will benefit from eating plenty of calcium-rich dairy foods.

CHILDHOOD

Just like adults, growing children need a balanced diet that includes a variety of nutritious foods. Children may have insatiable appetites during a growth spurt but a more limited appetite in between spurts.

Nutrients of concern: Calcium is especially important during childhood as the body's skeleton develops. Picky eating or eating a diet with little variety can make it harder for kids to get the vitamins, minerals, protein, and dietary fiber that they need.

INFANCY

Newborns need feeding regularly in order to meet their high calorific needs. Breast milk and infant formula are the best sources of nutrition, providing not only adequate calories, but also proteins, fats, carbohydrates, and essential vitamins and minerals.

Nutrients of concern: To prevent vitamin K deficiency bleeding, every baby is given a shot of vitamin K at birth. Exclusively breastfed babies may also need a vitamin D supplement. Most experts recommend 200 to 400 IU (5–10 mcg) per day of vitamin D for infants until they receive enough formula in addition to breastmilk to meet their needs, or until they start to eat solid foods that provide enough vitamin D.

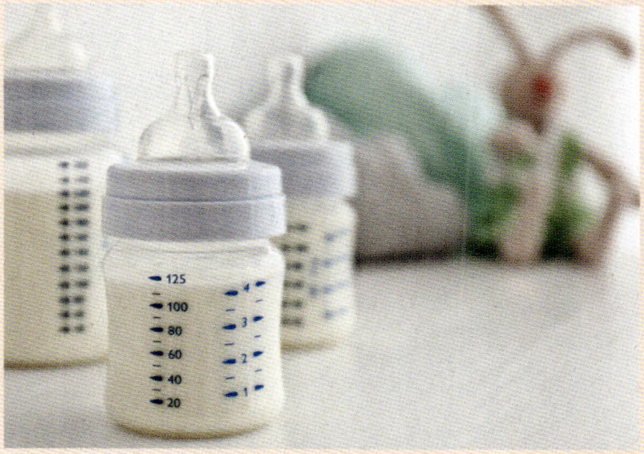

Formula milk is fortified with vitamin D.

DID YOU KNOW?

Babies have the highest caloric needs per unit of body weight than any other stage in the life cycle.

NUTRIENT TIPS

Children prefer sweet tastes and tend to be more sensitive to bitter tastes until adolescence and sometimes even into adulthood. If you hated Brussels sprouts, broccoli, or dark chocolate as a kid, give them another try as an adult. Adults have more tolerance to bitter foods and can develop a liking to them. You can use cooking techniques such as pickling, roasting, and braising to improve the tastes of some bitter foods.

ADOLESCENCE

Growth and puberty during the preteen and teenage years typically requires more calories per day than any other time of life. (Infants need the most calories relative to body weight, but growing teens need the most total daily calories.) Eating a nutritious diet is of utmost importance during adolescence, but as teenagers become more autonomous in their food choices, snacks, treats, and fast foods may take precedence over more nutritious foods. In addition, disordered eating may start to develop during this stage of the life cycle.

Nutrients of concern: Boys tend to need more calories than girls, while girls require more iron than boys due to the onset of their periods. Calcium and vitamin D continue to be nutrients of the greatest importance during this time to build healthy bones.

ADULTHOOD

After adolescence, energy needs start to decrease. As young adults transition into the workforce, they may start to cook more meals at home and/or have more control over the foods they purchase and eat. This can lead to more healthful eating, or on the other hand, an increased consumption of restaurant and packaged foods, alcohol, and caffeine. Eating a nutritious diet continues to be important throughout adulthood, especially in relation to health maintenance and disease prevention. Dietary habits in young adulthood may increase or decrease the risk of developing health conditions later in life.

Nutrients of concern: Adults may exceed calorie and sodium needs, while also getting too much added sugar and not enough fluids and fiber.

OLDER ADULTHOOD

Elderly individuals typically need fewer calories compared to earlier life stages, since they usually exercise less and have less muscle mass. However, they still need similar or higher amounts of certain micronutrients.

Nutrients of concern: Older adults require more calcium and vitamin D to support optimal bone health. They may also need more vitamin B12, due to malabsorption and other issues (see also page 56). Constipation is common in older adulthood, and thus it's important to drink enough water and consume enough fiber.

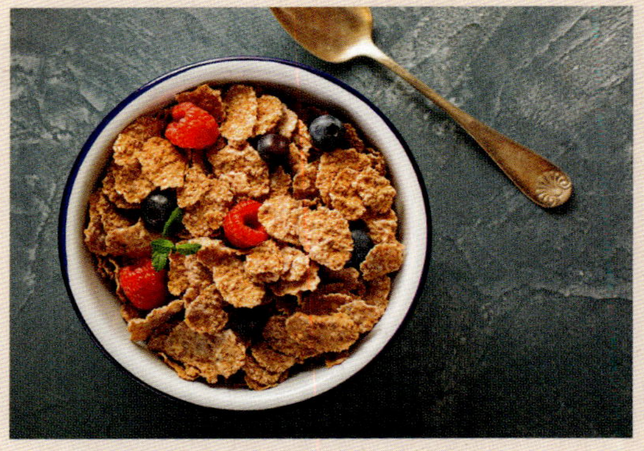

Eating fortified cereals with vitamin D fortified milk, helps maintain bone health, while providing dietary fiber.

A MINDFUL APPROACH TO SUPPLEMENTS

As we age, it becomes more tempting to turn to supplements. Before taking any type of supplement—whether a vitamin or mineral, or any of those discussed on pages 142–45)—remember to ask yourself if, and why, you need a particular product. Clever marketing may make it seem like a certain pill is a miracle worker or must-have product. But before you dive in and make a purchase, do your due diligence in researching the product and brand. Are there studies to back the proposed claims on the label? And even more importantly, do you actually need or desire the effects that the supplements promise?

[HEALTHY EATING SCHEDULE]

It's time to put your newfound knowledge of vitamins and minerals into action! Remember, it's best to meet your nutrient needs naturally, through foods, rather than supplements, and eating a varied diet will ensure that you do just that.

On the following pages, you will find a sample healthy eating schedule that will help you visualize the types of foods you should be incorporating into your meals over the course of a week, in order to get enough vitamins and minerals. Each day of the week is covered, along with a suggestion for breakfast, lunch, dinner, and a snack. The main nutrients for each meal are also listed for easy reference. Take a photo of the sample meals or bookmark the pages to refer to throughout the week.

There are options that include both plant and animal sources of each nutrient, but keep in mind that there are many other nutritious foods that are not listed.

If you tend to eat less of a certain food one week and more the next—such as leafy greens or nuts and seeds—that's OK! Adequate nutrition is more than the sum of its parts, and there's always room to increase or decrease your intake of certain foods if needed. Nutrition recommendations, such as the RDAs and AIs, tend to focus on daily needs for vitamins and minerals. However, it's not necessary to obsess over meeting these exact numbers every day. Instead, focus on getting enough nutrients over the course of a week, spread out over seven days' worth of meals.

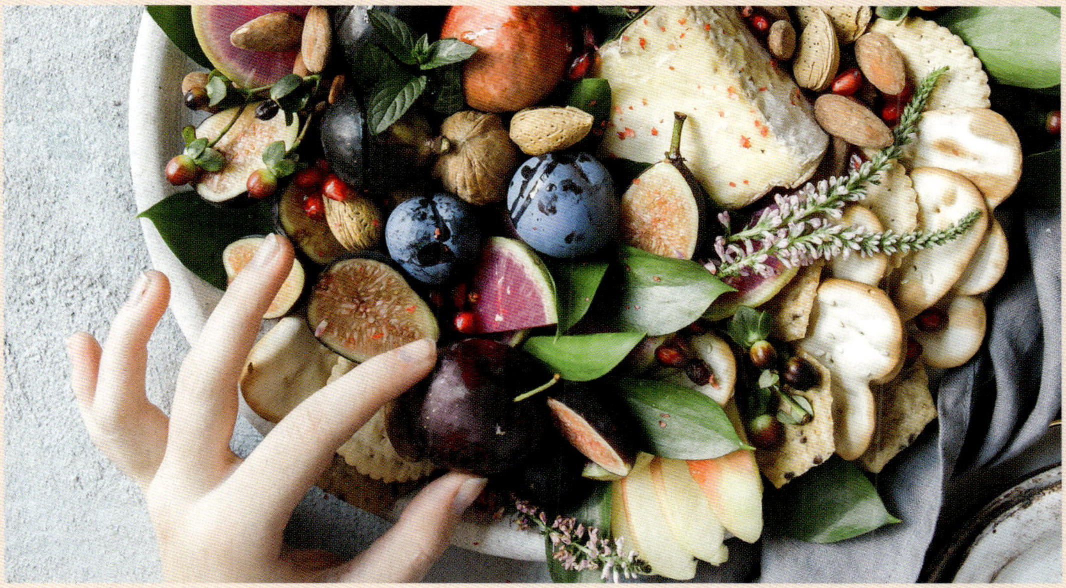

AT-A-GLANCE GUIDE FOR HEALTHY MEALS

	MONDAY	TUESDAY	WEDNESDAY
BREAKFAST	Omelet with sautéed mushrooms and shredded cheese, orange	Greek yogurt with chia seeds and cantaloupe	Poached eggs with whole wheat toast and avocado
Essential vitamins and minerals covered	Vitamins C, D, and B3, choline, calcium	Vitamins A, B2, and C, calcium	Vitamins D and B12, potassium, molybdenum
LUNCH	Kale salad with shredded turkey	Burrito bowl with brown rice, avocado, black beans, and salsa	Tomato soup and grilled cheese
Essential vitamins and minerals covered	Vitamins A, K, B6, and B12, chromium	Vitamins E, B3, B5, and B9, magnesium	Vitamin A, calcium, potassium
DINNER	Salmon, baked potato, asparagus	Chicken breast, sautéed spinach, buttered noodles	Tofu stir-fry with broccoli, peppers, and peanut sauce
Essential vitamins and minerals covered	Vitamin B9, phosphorus, potassium, iodine	Vitamins K and B12, iron	Vitamins C and K, biotin, chromium, iron
SNACKS	Brazil nuts, dried apricots	Dark chocolate, banana and peanut butter	Pineapple and pecans in yogurt
Essential vitamins and minerals covered	Vitamin A, selenium	Biotin, magnesium, potassium, molybdenum	Vitamin C, calcium, manganese,

THURSDAY	FRIDAY	SATURDAY	SUNDAY
Oatmeal, pears, cinnamon, pumpkin seeds	English muffin with peanut butter, blueberries	Overnight oats with shredded carrots, pecans, and coconut	Swiss chard frittata with goat cheese, fortified orange juice
Vitamins B1, B2, and B3, zinc	Vitamins A and B9, chromium, copper	Vitamins A and E, manganese	Vitamins D, B9, and K, choline, calcium
Hamburger on a bed of lettuce with tomato and onion, sliced apples	Grain bowls with quinoa, chickpeas, parsley, feta cheese in lemon juice and olive oil	Lentil soup with arugula salad	Chicken salad sandwich, raspberries
Vitamins K and B12, iron	Vitamins E, K, and B6, iron	Vitamin B9, magnesium, iron	Vitamins B3, B6, and biotin, iron
Chili-stuffed sweet potatoes with shredded cheese	Pork chop, sautéed apples and onions, mashed potatoes	Shrimp scampi pasta with zucchini	Eggplant Parmesan, roasted green beans
Vitamins A, B5, and B9, biotin, calcium	Vitamins B1, B12, and C, iron	Vitamin B12, phosphorus, iodine, selenium	Vitamin B6, potassium, chromium, manganese
Cashew nuts and dried cherries	Carrot sticks and guacamole	Vitamin D fortified milk and cookies	Air popped popcorn with nutritional yeast
Vitamin C, copper	Vitamins A, E, and B5	Vitamins B2 and D, calcium	Vitamin B12, magnesium

[INDEX]

[ACKNOWLEDGMENTS]

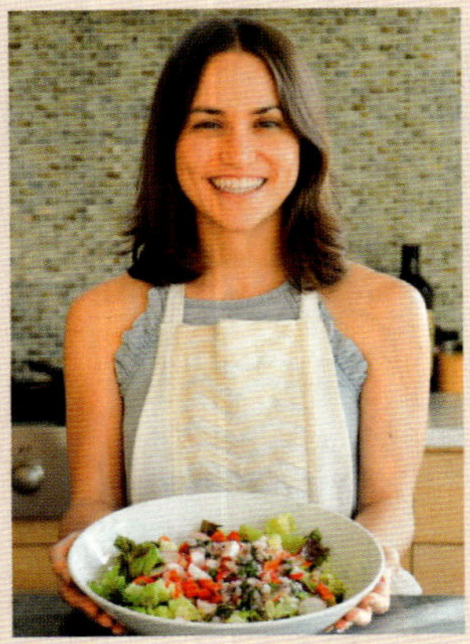

ABOUT THE AUTHOR

Lizzie Streit, MS, RDN, LD is a registered dietitian, nutrition writer, and recipe developer with a master's degree in human nutrition. She is the creator of It's a Veg World After All® and author of *Vegetable Cookbook for Vegetarians: 200 Recipes from Artichoke to Zucchini*. Through her published works and recipes, she is devoted to helping others achieve and maintain good health by increasing their knowledge of nutrition and cooking skills. When she's not in the kitchen, Lizzie enjoys exploring the local food scene in Minneapolis, exercising around the lakes and trails, and experimenting with her backyard vegetable garden. To see more of her work, visit **itsavegworldafterall.com**.

PICTURE CREDITS

t = top; c = center; b = bottom; l = left; r = right

Unsplash
Pages 2, 9, 155: Brooke Lark; 4–5: Yash Bhoir; 6: Tanaphong Toochinda; 12–13: Vanesa Conunaese; 14: LUM3N; 17t: Epicurrence; 17cl: Sam Abtahi; 17bl: Juan Gomez; 17br: Brad Stallcup; 18: Sarah Gualtieri; 21t: Micheile Henderson; 21bl: Alice Pasqual; 25cr: Remi Yuan; 26: Jo Sonn; 29bl, 127t: Eaters Collective; 29cr: Ronit Shaked; 30: Alexander Mils; 36: Svitlana; 37t, 81bl: Ellieelien; 37bl, 45t, 49bl, 89t, 99t, 132–133: Ella Olsson; 37cr, 141: Stephanie Studer; 37br: Chad Montano; 45bl: Andrei; 46: Charles Deluvio; 49t, 134, 140, 149: Monika Grabkowska; 49cr: cleo stracuzza; 53bl: Carly Jane; 53cr: LYFE Fuel; 57cl: Mc Jefferson Agloro; 60: Katarzyna Grabowska; 61cr: Gabriel Gurrola; 62: Jiangxulei1990; 65bl: Joseph Gonzalez; 65cr: Sebastian Coman Photography; 69bl: Jennifer Schmidt; 69cr: Tetiana Bykovets; 70–71: Niclas Illg; 75bl, 148bl: Anh Nguyen; 75cr: Brenda Godinez; 76: Vince Lee; 81cr: Charisse Kenion; 85t: Amber Engle; 85bl: Jenn Kosar; 89bl: Nathan Dumlao; 89cr: Megan Markham; 96: Gaby Yerden; 103t: Charlotte Coneybeer; 104: Joanna Kosinska; 107bl: Anna Wlodarczyk; 107br: Deryn Macey; 111bl: Cody Chan; 112: Anshu A; 115bl: Sandi Benedicta; 119bl: American Heritage Chocolate; 123t: Hari Nandakumar; 124: Vino Li; 131bl: dimitri.photography; 135t: Harris; 135b: Nicholas Barbaros; 138cl: Caroline Atwood; 138br: Jakub Kapusnak; 139: Davies Designs Studio; 143t: Shannon Milling; 143b: Manki Kim; 146: Carissa Gan; 147: David Todd McCarty; 148cr: Nadine Primeau; 150: Yulia Khlebnikova; 151: Neha Deshmukh; 152: Duarte Nunes.

Shutterstock
Pages 7, 33t: Ekaterina Kondratova; 21cr: Maslova Valentina; 22: j.chizhe; 25t: zarzamora; 25bl: Ratov Maxim; 28: Gayvoronskaya_Yana; 29t: nesavinov; 32: mama_mia; 33bl: kibokal; 33cr, 85br, 115t: Kiian Oksana; 34: Dasha_Romanova; 38: photopixel; 41t: Magdanatka; 41bl: AnikonaAnn; 41cr: SosnaRadosna; 42: lesyakikh; 45cr: Pinkyone; 50, 111cr: MasterQ; 53t: Sergii Gnatiuk; 54: Viktor1; 57t: Joshua Resnick; 57bl: SUPERGAL; 57br: Ruslan Mitin; 58: beton studio; 61t: EvennreisCat; 61bl: ShotnCut; 65t, 69br: Anna_Pustynnikova; 66: virtu studio; 69t, 115cr, 123bl, 154: Elena Veselova; 72: Alexander Prokopenko; 75t: SEE D JAN; 78, 127bl: Letterberry; 81t: Magdanatka; 82: MaraZe; 86: Jagoda Przybyla; 90: bogdandimages; 93t: Melica; 93bl: Marian Weyo; 93cr: Jade Y; 94, 103cr: New Africa; 99bl: Vezzani Photography; 99cr: Robby Cyron Photography; 100: Nina Firsova; 103bl: pilipphoto 103 bl; 107t: Amarita; 108: Nickola_Che; 111t: ILEISH ANNA; 116: 5 second Studio; 119t: Regreto; 119cr: I Ketut Tamba Budiarsana; 120: FuzullHanum; 123cr: DiAnna Paulk; 127br: HandmadePictures; 128: Javier Somoza; 131t: gowithstock; 131br: Jiri Hera; 136: Denise I Johnson; 144: Pixel-Shot; 145: LukHt; 153t: nevodka; 153cr: Africa Studio.

Page 160: Allie Bornstein Photography